D1028011

How to have a baby

a baby

And Still Live in the Real World

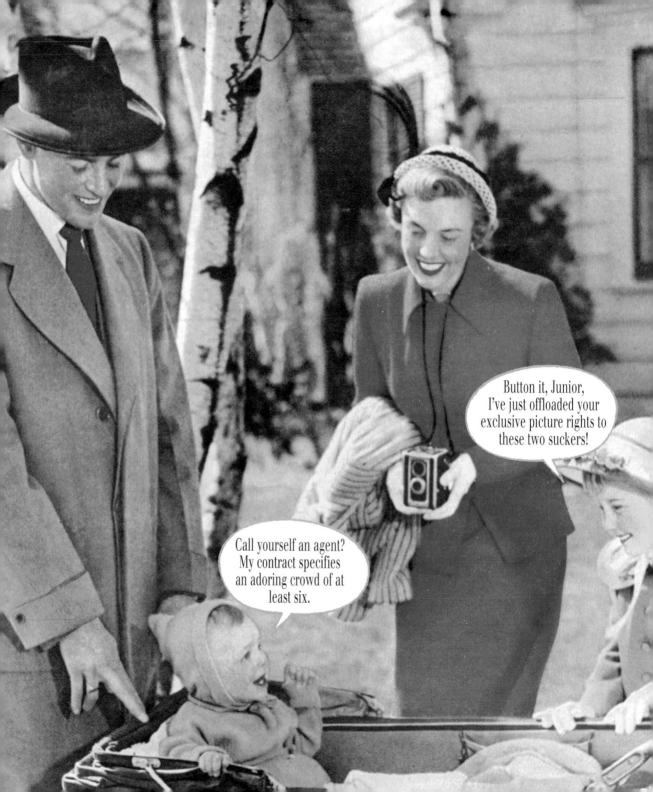

NEW HANOVER COUNTY
PUBLIC LIBRARY
201 CHESTNUT STREET
WILMINGTON, NC 28401

How to have a baby

And Still Live in the Real World

Jane Symons

Consulting Editor: Dr. Gila Leiter

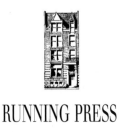

RUNNING PRESS

Text © 2003 The Ivy Press Limited
First published in the United States in 2003 by Running Press Book Publishers
All rights reserved under the Pan-American and International Copyright Conventions
Printed in China

This book may not be reproduced in whole or in part, in any form or by
any means, electronic or mechanical, including photocopying, recording, or
by any information storage and retrieval system now known or hereafter
invented, without written permission from the publisher.

9   8   7   6   5   4   3   2   1
Digit on the right indicates the number of this printing

Library of Congress Cataloging-in-Publication Number 2002108895

ISBN 0-7624-1447-2

This book was created by
THE IVY PRESS LTD
The Old Candlemakers,
Lewes, East Sussex BN7 2NZ

CREATIVE DIRECTOR *Peter Bridgewater*

PUBLISHER *Sophie Collins*

EDITORIAL DIRECTOR *Steve Luck*

ART DIRECTOR *Clare Barber*

DESIGN MANAGER *Tony Seddon*

SENIOR PROJECT EDITOR *Caroline Earle*

DESIGNER *Kevin Knight*

ILLUSTRATIONS *Moira Wills*

This book may be ordered by mail from the publisher. Please include $2.50 for postage and handling.
But try your bookstore first!

Running Press Book Publishers
125 South Twenty-second Street
Philadelphia, Pennsylvania 19103-4399

Visit us on the web!
www.runningpress.com

CONTENTS

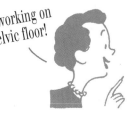

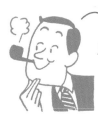

❋ I'm working on my pelvic floor!

❋ That's great honey, I'll get my hammer and nails!

Sickness, mood swings, fatigue ...can't wait!

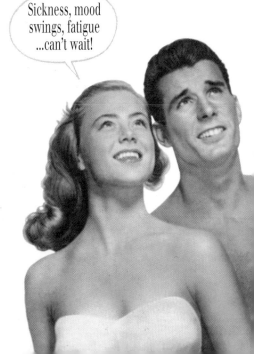

INTRODUCTION WELCOME TO THE CLUB!

Pregnancy is the ultimate lifechanger. A new job, a new town, a new man—these are minor ripples on the Richter scale compared with the major earthquake of impending motherhood. You had better start getting used to the idea of change now, because once you've seen the thin line that screams "Positive!" on your pregnancy test, life will never be the same again. Your body will change, your priorities will change, and some of your relationships will probably change, too.

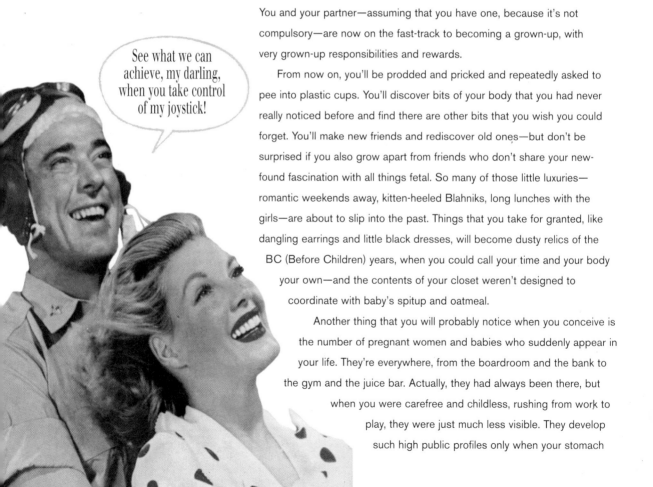

See what we can achieve, my darling, when you take control of my joystick!

You and your partner—assuming that you have one, because it's not compulsory—are now on the fast-track to becoming a grown-up, with very grown-up responsibilities and rewards.

From now on, you'll be prodded and pricked and repeatedly asked to pee into plastic cups. You'll discover bits of your body that you had never really noticed before and find there are other bits that you wish you could forget. You'll make new friends and rediscover old ones—but don't be surprised if you also grow apart from friends who don't share your new-found fascination with all things fetal. So many of those little luxuries—romantic weekends away, kitten-heeled Blahniks, long lunches with the girls—are about to slip into the past. Things that you take for granted, like dangling earrings and little black dresses, will become dusty relics of the BC (Before Children) years, when you could call your time and your body your own—and the contents of your closet weren't designed to coordinate with baby's spitup and oatmeal.

Another thing that you will probably notice when you conceive is the number of pregnant women and babies who suddenly appear in your life. They're everywhere, from the boardroom and the bank to the gym and the juice bar. Actually, they had always been there, but when you were carefree and childless, rushing from work to play, they were just much less visible. They develop such high public profiles only when your stomach starts out on its own, similarly impressive, march to prominence. As your belly swells, you'll also find that personal space has a funny habit of shrinking. All sorts of people will try to pat you on the belly or offer advice—whether you want it, or not.

So, welcome to the club. That's what parenthood is all about—it gives you a lifetime pass to the biggest, and some would say the best and most influential, club on earth. In the next nine months, you'll go boldly where so many have gone before you, and discover that every second person has their own toe-curlingly gruesome pregnancy/birth story to tell. Casual acquaintances and complete strangers will suddenly feel compelled to share their most intimate gynecological secrets with you while waiting in the line at the ATM. Whether it's the waters that broke during a pitch for a business plan that had a longer gestation than an elephant, or the marathon labor from hell, there's likely to be no escape until you've heard every last graphic detail.

You'll hear a lot of other stories, too. Some will make you laugh, some will make you think, and some will provide glittering gems of advice. As a mom who's also a health writer, I've heard more stories than most, and in the course of writing this book I've also talked to dozens of nurse-midwives, obstetricians, and researchers to sort out the facts from the fiction. But most of all, I've talked to moms—and it's their stories, and sanity-saving tips, that I would like to share with you.

Knowing what hormones can do to a girl's brain, I won't claim to answer every single question that could come up in the next nine months, but I will cover all of the big ones. At times, this might make pregnancy sound scarier than a dinner date with Hannibal Lecter, but don't panic. Although there are lots of things that can go wrong, they very rarely do. And if you're one of the one or two percent that stuff happens to, it's good to know that you're not alone. Along the way,

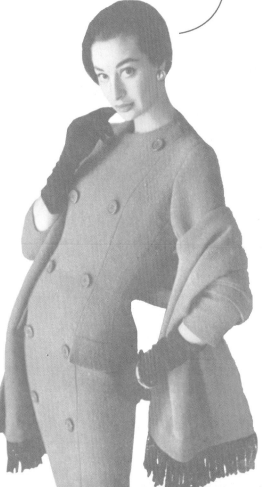

✳ Take a good look, buster: that's the last you'll see of these hip bones for the next nine months.

I'll also try to answer quite a few of the questions that your mother or doctor might forget to mention. More importantly, I'll share the experiences of real women in real situations and, I hope, bring a little light relief, because there are going to be times when you'll need it!

The first rule of pregnancy is that there aren't any rules. Sure, there are plenty of commonsense guidelines, which you'll find throughout this book, and you should always follow medical advice. But hey, this is the real world, and in the real world we're not all perfect—sometimes moms-in-the-making have an occasional cigarette or glass of wine, sometimes we eat too much junk food, and sometimes we don't get enough exercise. That's life—at least, that's life in the world that I inhabit. When I was pregnant with my first child, I began to wonder whether pregnancy gurus lived in the same world. Second time around, I began to wonder whether they lived on the same planet. It might be life, but as Mr. Spock would say, "Not as we know it."

So who are "we"? Call us the mom's club, call us sisters, call us whatever you like—we've probably heard it before. "We" are moms. And we know that no two pregnancies are the same, and no two women have exactly the same views of motherhood. Even if you're reading this as a refresher and you've been there, done that (and have a closet full of baggy T-shirts to prove it), you'll probably find that pregnancy can be very different the second, or third, time around.

The second rule of pregnancy is that it rarely goes by the book—not even this one—and there are all sorts of pleasant, and sometimes not so pleasant, surprises in store from your body and your baby. Blame it on hormones—in fact, over the next nine-and-a-half months, you can blame hormones for just about everything: tiredness,

OK Blanche, congratulations already—do we really have to sing the Hallelujah Chorus?

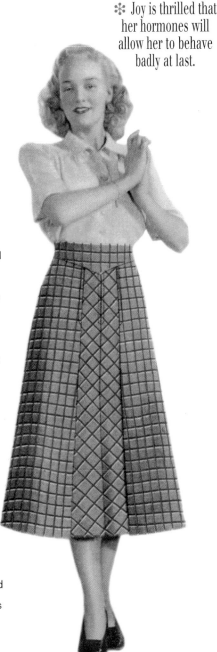

❋ Joy is thrilled that her hormones will allow her to behave badly at last.

elation, mood swings, feeling fabulous, insatiable sex drive, complete loss of libido, forgetfulness, and food cravings. Those are just a few of the side effects of the heady cocktail of body chemicals that is beginning to slosh around your bloodstream.

So why on earth does any sane woman set herself up for all of this—let alone go back for seconds, thirds, and sometimes double helpings? Some people believe that pregnancy shrinks the female brain—which probably explains all those times you'll leave your sports bag at work and take your briefcase to yoga—but there's a lot more to it than a few absent brain cells. Babies are continually demanding, completely selfish, utterly exhausting, and simply wonderful. They can reduce you to tears of frustration or sobs of helpless laughter. Their first smile is ecstasy, their first tooth will probably be hell. Babies are a bit like nuclear physics—a tiny clump of cells will mushroom into something that will change your world forever.

Labor wards can have strange effects on people, too. The natural health earth mother can suddenly forget all about yoga and flower remedies and start screaming for drugs, lots of drugs, NOW! The princess who always thought that she was far too delicate to push may discover that a TENS machine isn't so bad after all, and find herself holding a baby before she can utter the words "elective Cesarean."

Only one thing is guaranteed: the rollercoaster that is pregnancy and childbirth is only just beginning. From now on, you will experience one helluva learning curve after another as you embark on the ride of a lifetime. It's full of thrills and spills, but having kids is *the* life experience.

And even if you've been there before, childbirth can still come as a surprise. There's many a second- or third-time mom who goes into labor and suddenly realizes: "Omigod, now I remember what it feels like!" Sure it hurts —like hell—but having babies hurts a whole lot less when you go into labor with information, support, and realistic expectations.

Finding out!

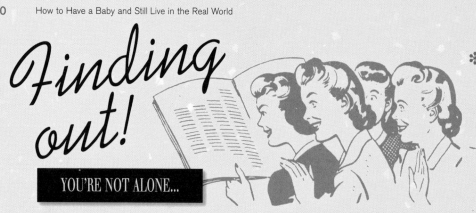

❋ Her classmates were amazed that tomboy Thelma had made motherhood at last.

YOU'RE NOT ALONE...

The odds of getting pregnant make winning the lottery look like a pushover. According to the World Health Organization, there are 42,000 million episodes of sex per year—that's more than 1,300 ejaculations per second. However, all that sex results in just nine babies being born every two seconds, so to beat the odds that's a heck of a lot of practice rounds to get in!

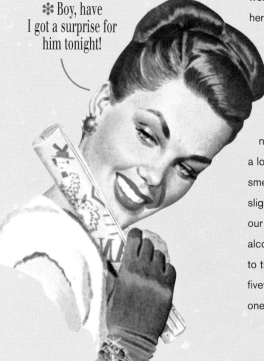

❋ Boy, have I got a surprise for him tonight!

A missed period is the most obvious clue that you're in a motherly way, but it is not the only one. Also, this doesn't always happen when you conceive: a woman can be pregnant but still get a very light bleed around the time that her next period is due. This "period" will be lighter and shorter, which is why your doctor will be more interested in the date of your last "normal" period. As a general rule, conception occurs about two weeks before you actually miss a period, which is why some women suspect that something's up before they're even late. Common clues include breast tenderness, mood swings, headaches, and bloating—nothing new to PMS veterans. Other clues are a bit more of a giveaway. You pee a lot. At the same time, joy of joys, you may be constipated. Your sense of smell suddenly rivals that of Lassie the Wonder Dog. There may be an odd, slightly metallic taste in your mouth (familiar to those of us who used to suck our paintbrushes in first grade). You suddenly lose all interest in coffee, alcohol, and cigarettes. You have increased vaginal discharge. You feel tired to the point of utter exhaustion—but if you have just negotiated a difficult fiveway contract, or worked three nightshifts back to back, or ridden herd on one or more preschool children, how surprising is that?

Don't worry if you haven't noticed any of these symptoms. Every woman and pregnancy is different, and will produce slightly different levels of hormones. All these changes have more to do with how quickly the chemicals kick in, and how easily your body adapts to them, than your powers of observation.

Testing times

You may be convinced that you have conceived, but you will still need official confirmation. There are two ways to confirm you're pregnant: a blood test or a urine test. They're both looking for a hormone called human chorionic gonadotrophin (HCG), which is made by the developing placenta to stimulate the production of estrogen and progesterone (*see pages 29–31*).

Blood tests are very accurate; they can detect very low levels of HCG and can be done as early as seven days after ovulation, long before your period is even overdue. Another plus is that they indicate how much HCG is present. This can help your doctor or nurse-midwife to accurately pinpoint your dates; in the early stages of pregnancy, HCG levels double every couple of days and peak between the seventh and tenth week. The downsides of a blood test are that you can't do it yourself, and it takes a few days for the results to come through.

Urine tests that you can do at home give almost instant results, but there is no point doing one until the first day your period is due. If you do the test too early, you'll be flushing money down the toilet because chances are there won't be enough pregnancy hormones in your system to show up.

If you do them at the right time, and follow the directions, home tests are pretty accurate. There are lots of different pregnancy tests on the market, and they all work in much the same way: by using a plastic dipstick to check whether there's any HCG in your pee. The amount of HCG that can be detected varies from kit to kit, and this is usually shown on the package. Either way, the lower the number, the more sensitive the test.

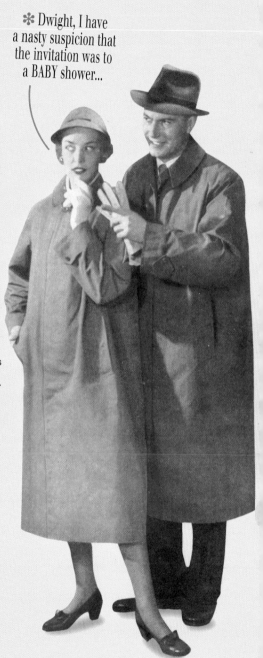

✳ Dwight, I have a nasty suspicion that the invitation was to a BABY shower...

WATER DIVINING
TESTS AND DATES

It's not essential, but it's best to do the home pregnancy test first thing in the morning, because this is when your HCG levels will be at their highest. If you drop a cup full of urine in your excitement, at least you will be in the tranquil confines of your own bathroom. If you are doing the test during the day, make sure that you haven't had a pee for at least four hours and don't try to drink lots of water beforehand, because this will only dilute the amount of HCG in your pee. The easiest way to do one of these tests is to hold the popsicle stick in your urine stream. If this sounds a bit too hands-on, use a clean paper cup or beaker to collect a midstream sample (i.e., not the first few drops, and not the last ones, either). Then dip the stick into the sample for a few seconds. (Now is the time to get used to peeing onto small sticks and into tiny receptacles with pinpoint accuracy, because you'll be doing this with tedious regularity throughout your pregnancy.) Most pregnancy kits have a test window that changes color to confirm a result, and the directions will say how long it should take for something to happen. This is rarely more than a few minutes, and may be only a matter of seconds, but it will probably feel like a lifetime.

Are you sure this is the right sort of test probe, Captain?

If you're doing the test at work, here are some tips on doing it without the entire office discovering your little secret. Try to avoid the postlunch rush to the toilet. If the office busybody happens to be parked by the door, buy a spare pair of pantyhose and slip the pregnancy test into the same bag: it will disguise the kit and provides a smokescreen if he or she notices that you've been awhile (this is not the time to say you're feeling a bit unwell, even if you are). Use a stall that has one of those chemical bins for pads and tampons so that you can set the test down flat on the lid (someone might spot it if you use the floor). Most of all, try not to scream "Yippee!" or "Oh my God!" when you see the result.

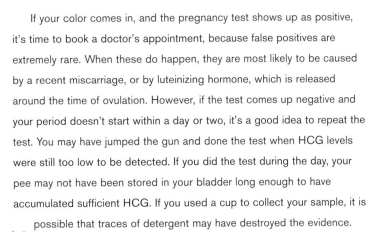

USE YOUR EDD

The date every mom-to-be is most interested in is the expected date of delivery (EDD). It's easy enough to work out: just count 40 weeks from the first day of your last period. For instance, if that was January 1, your baby is due on October 8. But remember, this isn't mail order and there are no guaranteed delivery dates.

Yippee!

If your color comes in, and the pregnancy test shows up as positive, it's time to book a doctor's appointment, because false positives are extremely rare. When these do happen, they are most likely to be caused by a recent miscarriage, or by luteinizing hormone, which is released around the time of ovulation. However, if the test comes up negative and your period doesn't start within a day or two, it's a good idea to repeat the test. You may have jumped the gun and done the test when HCG levels were still too low to be detected. If you did the test during the day, your pee may not have been stored in your bladder long enough to have accumulated sufficient HCG. If you used a cup to collect your sample, it is possible that traces of detergent may have destroyed the evidence. Other factors that can interfere with pregnancy tests include the hormones used in fertility treatments.

Blind dates

When it comes to age, it's easier to pin down a fortysomething female than the average embryo, which is why pregnancy officially begins on the first day of your last menstrual period (LMP); it's the only date that you can really be sure of. In reality, you won't have conceived until a couple of weeks later, sometime around the middle of your menstrual cycle, when you hit peak fertility and an egg is released. This means that what your doctor calls the sixth week of pregnancy is more likely to be four weeks from conception. For simplicity, we'll use the LMP calculation when talking about pregnancy dates. This arithmetic explains why a baby can arrive two weeks early, or two weeks late, and still be considered on time, and why we talk of pregnancy lasting nine months when it's 9.3 months by this calculation (*see box above* for details on working out your expected delivery date). This may sound like splitting hairs, but talk to anyone who's done it recently and she'll tell you that the last 0.3 of a month feels like a year.

CHAIN REACTIONS

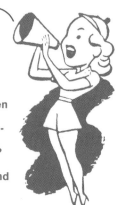

Hey girls, it's positive!

So, you've done the test and discovered that one of your partner's sperm has beaten the biological odds and scored a touchdown. Gulp! You may find yourself double- and triple-checking the pregnancy test kit, or asking your doctor, "Are you sure? Could the lab have gotten the results mixed up? Maybe they got the wrong rabbit? And while we're at it, what do bunnies have to do with making babies?"

❋ After their phone was cut off, Brad and Janet simply semaphored the good news to the family.

Actually, they don't use rabbits any more. Even when they did, contrary to modern myth, all the rabbits died. It goes back to the 1920s, when someone discovered that injecting urine from a pregnant woman into a female rabbit caused it to develop growths on its ovaries—but the only way to find out whether they were there was to kill the rabbit and dissect it.

Seeing a pregnancy test, *your* pregnancy test, change color before your eyes may leave you speechless with delight. Madeleine, a 24-year-old first-timer says, "I felt like a cat with a saucer of cream, I couldn't say a word, I just couldn't stop smiling." Or speechless with emotion—Celia, who's 38 and already a partner in her law firm, says, "I'm usually really organized and in control, but when the test came up positive, my mind went crazy. I can't remember when I ever felt so excited and confused, all at the same time."

Or perhaps you were already so convinced that you had conceived that the confirmation came as no surprise. Sally, who is 29 and a nurse-midwife, says: "I knew that the test would be positive. All day long I'd been talking to women who'd just learned that they were pregnant and they kept mentioning things that were ringing big bells—having a funny taste in your mouth, going off coffee, sore tits. It wasn't a planned pregnancy and when I saw the result I was numb, I didn't know what to think. At first, I felt guilty that I wasn't delighted."

All of these reactions are perfectly normal, so don't beat yourself up if you're feeling more shocked than overjoyed. You'll probably ricochet through the emotional alphabet, from anticipation to Zenlike calm and back again to anxiety. There are no rules to the way women feel when they discover that they are pregnant, and a whole host of different factors come into play—the stability of your relationship, whether or not you have a relationship; your finances; your health; your family history; and even the size of your apartment. Nothing prepares you for the flood of emotions or mindnumbing uncertainty that can follow. You may be elated and excited, or you may feel like a frightened rabbit caught in car headlights. You may feel tranquil, or you may be completely terrified. You may be nervous, or nauseous with anticipation—or is that morning sickness? More on that on pages 36–39.

Keeping mum

You might not want to tell anyone else for a little bit, not even your partner. Sometimes women just want to enjoy their big secret for a while. If it is a second or third child, you may find yourself rummaging through your closets for the tiny shirts your now gigantic toddler(s) once wore and staring wildly at them, handfuls of tissues at the ready. All those memories will come flooding back to you (and I mean all). You might prefer to keep the news just between you and your partner for the first three months. There are two advantages to this: he will have an explanation for your mood swings (another, almost universal, symptom of pregnancy); and you might avoid the pain of having to explain a miscarriage to friends and family. An estimated 14–18 percent of all pregnancies end in miscarriages, and most of these take place within the first 12 weeks. Miscarriage is usually caused by what physicians call the nonviability of the embryo—which is a way of saying it's really for the best.

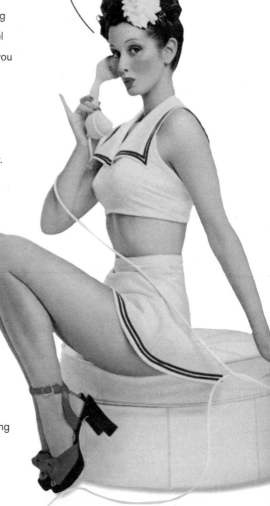

❋ Momma, that divine little two-piece you made me just got way too small.

Once you decide to spread the news, be prepared for a tsunami of advice and anecdote. The upside is that, with your first pregnancy, you join a worldwide club you didn't know existed; the downside is that every member will want to tell you about it. Pay close attention to women who have produced a baby recently—they're the ones who are most likely to offer useful tips. Antenatal and birth practices change frequently, and your mother's recollections may not be very relevant (although it's always nice to be told how lovely you were).

What, when, why....

Whatever your reaction, we have found that there is one thing that most moms-to-be have in common: questions, questions, and more questions. What's good/bad for my baby? What will my partner think? Do I need a partner? What should I eat? Can I color my hair? Should I stop drinking coffee? Why don't I like coffee any more? Should I use the computer? Is the microwave safe? What was that I heard about cats? Do I have to give up sex? Will everything be OK? What's happening to my body?

Write down specific questions you want to ask, and then work out who is the best person to answer them: your doctor, your nurse-midwife, your partner, a girlfriend who's just had a baby, your mother, your mother-in-law, or a newfound friend in an Internet chatroom. The sooner you get into the habit of writing lists and checking off items, the easier it will be later on: once the pregnancy hormones kick in, these scraps of paper often become lifelines that keep you moored to the shores of sanity. Later on in the pregnancy, while you're waiting for action, it can also be a laugh to look back on these early thoughts and see how far you, and your baby, have come.

ESSENTIALS

THE NAME GAME

By the time your fertilized egg has divided into enough cells to reach double figures, it's known as a morula. By around seven days after conception, when it's grown to around 150 cells, it's called a blastocyst. This has two distinct sections: one becomes the baby and the other grows into the placenta and amniotic sac. By week five, it has multiplied into millions of cells, looks like a tiny tadpole, and goes by the name "embryo."

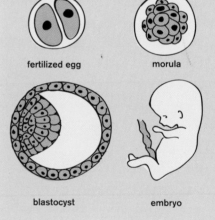

fertilized egg   morula

blastocyst   embryo

Multiplication and division

Strictly speaking, your baby isn't actually a baby at this stage of the game. In the first few weeks, it is little more than a clump of cells, and it goes by a variety of names, none of which are likely to appear on any family tree (*see diagram opposite*). At conception, your baby-to-be consists of a single cell containing all the genetic code that is needed to build a new person. About 12 hours later, this single cell splits into two. Another 12 hours later, two become four, and so on. Around the fifth week of pregnancy, the embryo develops three distinct sections: one becomes your baby's skin; the second becomes the muscles, bones, heart, kidneys, and reproductive organs; and the inner core develops into your baby's lungs, digestive system, and intestinal tract. So within ten weeks, that single cell has mushroomed into 6,000,000,000,000 (six trillion) cells. All of the organs have begun to form and a very basic heart is beating—with all that going on, it's no wonder you've been feeling tired.

Every time a cell splits, its characteristics and genetic information are reproduced. If something screws up this genetic code, the error is repeated every time a cell is reproduced. A cell error early in the pregnancy will be multiplied many millions of times over and may have catastrophic results. The critical period is between the fifth and tenth week of pregnancy, when the major organs are formed. If an error occurs later in the pregnancy, fewer cells will be damaged, but this can still cause serious problems.

By the tenth week of pregnancy (eight weeks from conception), the first bones have formed, and from this moment your doctor and nurse-midwife will use the term "fetus." Strictly speaking, your baby remains a fetus until it is born, but most moms-to-be prefer to call their bump a baby (although you'd be surprised at some of the other names we've heard, particularly once Junior starts kicking!).

❊ If she concentrated hard, Joan found she could almost hear the cells dividing.

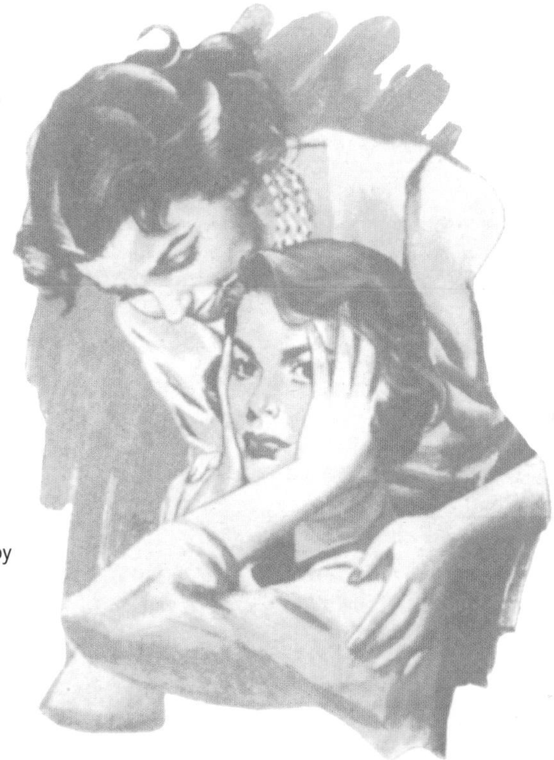

DOS AND DON'TS DURING PREGNANCY

The faster-than-a-speeding-bullet growth that takes place in the first few weeks after conception means that this early period is crucial to your baby's future health. In the real world, where most ZIP codes are still located, your diet and lifestyle might not have been perfect up to now. There's no point in beating yourself up over a tequila slammer or three, or because you are a stranger to leafy green vegetables. Guilt is no good for you, and no good for your baby.

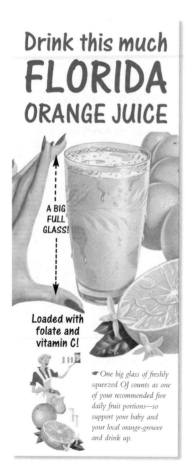

Drink this much
FLORIDA
ORANGE JUICE

A BIG FULL GLASS!

Loaded with folate and vitamin C!

☛ *One big glass of freshly squeezed OJ counts as one of your recommended five daily fruit portions—so support your baby and your local orange-grower and drink up.*

The past, as they say, is a foreign country, and your visa has just run out. But now that you have confirmed your pregnancy, there are no excuses. It may seem strange to be so cautious when you don't even have the beginnings of a bump, but there's plenty you can do now to improve the chances of a healthy baby and troublefree pregnancy.

Get fresh

Try to eat food that's fresh enough to remember where it came from and that still bears a passing resemblance to its original form—this doesn't usually come in a styrofoam box covered with corporate logos. Let's face it, you know you need lots of fruit and vegetables; plenty of carbohydrates, particularly less refined complex ones; and some form of protein, such as meat, fish, dairy products, soy, or legumes. Cut back on salt and saturated fats, and go easy on the sugar—and yes, that does include Oreos and ice cream.

Of all the nutrients that you need to know about, folate is the most crucial. Also called folic acid, this drives healthy cell division, which is why it is so important during pregnancy, particularly the early months. Low folate levels can lead to spinal deformities known as neural tube defects (NTDs). If you're not already taking a folate supplement, start right away on a 400-microgram daily dose. If you're one of those incredibly organized people (symptoms include filing your tax return on time and flossing after every meal) and are still at the planning stage, you should take a supplement for three months before conceiving. In fact, the U.S. Public Health Service advises all women who are capable of conception to make sure they get 400 micrograms of folic acid per day, just in case.

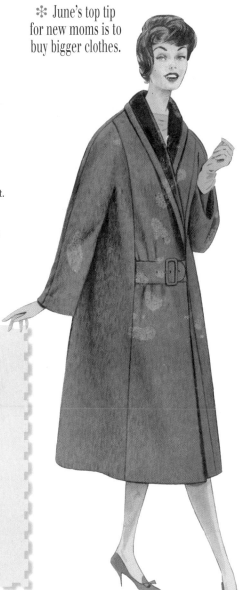

❊ June's top tip for new moms is to buy bigger clothes.

Bone up on calcium

Your baby needs calcium to build strong bones. If you're not providing enough from your diet, Junior will turn scavenger and start raiding the calcium you've been saving up for old age, so your own bone density will take a nosedive. Calcium deficiency is increasingly common, particularly among women who cut back on milk and dairy foods in order to lose weight. Dairy foods contain the highest concentrations of calcium (a pint of milk provides 90 percent of the Recommended Daily Intake). Other rich sources include sardines (with the bones) and collard greens. If you are a vegan, or have lactose intolerance, you can get calcium from soy, broccoli, oranges, almonds, Brazil nuts, molasses, sprouted seeds, and whole grains.

Iron files

Ask your mother if she took any supplements during pregnancy. She'll probably name iron, in foul-tasting, enormous pills. Cells need iron to generate energy, and it's a key ingredient in hemoglobin, the bell boy of the bloodstream, which carts oxygen around the body. Two out of every five women aged 18 to 34—the time when we're most likely to be having babies—have low iron. Vegetarians and people who don't eat much red meat are most at risk. This may

NTDs

Women who have a neural tube defect (NTD) themselves or have already conceived a child who has an NTD (this usually shows up on an ultrasound scan, see page 88), or who have a genetic deficiency in the enzyme that metabolizes folic acid, are advised to take higher doses of folic acid, up to 4,000 micrograms daily.

HOMEOPATHY

Homeopathic remedies are safe
so long as they are diluted above
24X (or 12C) since they contain
no discernable trace of active
ingredients. Nux vomica is
commonly recommended for
morning sickness and arnica can
be used for soreness and
bruising after delivery.

❋ Are you sure you don't want any? Well I guess I'll just have to force it down myself—I do need the calcium. And the jellybeans around my neck will make a great topping.

not be serious enough to make you anemic, but it does mean that you're not running on a full tank of gas. On the positive side, you're not losing iron through menstrual blood loss, and during pregnancy your body gets better at absorbing the stuff, so, contrary to what mom might say, you are unlikely to need an iron supplement in the early stages (and you can boost iron levels by drinking orange juice with iron-rich foods because vitamin C enhances iron absorption). In fact, there are arguments against taking iron at this stage because it slows up the absorption of zinc, which is more important early on.

Zinc on

Women who aren't getting enough zinc are more likely to miscarry, or have a low birthweight baby, which can have long-term health implications for your child. There is also increasing evidence that zinc deficiency increases the danger of birth defects involving the central nervous system. Deficiency is most likely if you don't eat much meat, are taking a high dose calcium supplement, have taken oral contraceptives for a long time, or work out a lot (because you literally sweat the stuff out). Natural zinc comes in much the same packaging as iron: high-protein meat and animal products.

Teratogens and other no-nos

The name for the no-nos that are known to cause fetal damage is "teratogen," an incredibly blunt bit of medical terminology that comes from the Greek word for monster—and you thought doctors were caring, sharing types! Your baby is most vulnerable to teratogens and other negative influences between the fifth and tenth week of pregnancy, but some teratogens remain dangerous throughout the pregnancy. Avoid them all, at all times.

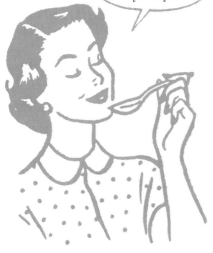

If I believe this extract of malt tastes yummy, it will taste yummy.

Prescription drugs that are known to cause problems include some of the ACE inhibitors used to treat high blood pressure, some epilepsy and blood-thinning drugs, and even some acne treatments. Don't kid yourself that herbal remedies are any safer. Some of the most toxic poisons known to man were cooked up by dear old Mother Nature. Some herbs induce uterine contractions or bleeding and should not be taken at any time in pregnancy. These include: arbor vitae, autumn crocus, bearberry, black cohosh, blue cohosh, broom, cotton root, feverfew, golden seal, greater celandine, juniper, life root, male fern, mistletoe, mugwort, nutmeg, pennyroyal, poke root, rue, southern wood, tansy, thuja, and wormwood.

The deal on drugs

There's nothing smart about taking recreational drugs, particularly when you're pregnant, but when an inner-city hospital anonymously tested newborns recently, it found that 40 percent had been exposed to drugs in the womb. Heroin and methadone cause stillbirth, mental retardation, prematurity, and low birthweight. Babies born to addicts are addicted, too. If you are hooked, at least try to get onto a methadone program. It's a little less damaging because your baby receives a regular, controlled, and clean dose.

Just one hit of crack or cocaine can cause serious damage, and babies born to abusers have to be weaned off the drugs. Marijuana is associated with low birthweight and prematurity, both of which increase the risk of long-term health problems for your child. LSD can cause miscarriage and chromosomal damage, and it's safe to assume that other hallucinogens will, too. Ecstasy hasn't been around long enough for us to assess its full impact, but animal studies show that it causes memory and learning impairments. Amphetamine, or speed, is linked to prematurity and may cause heart problems.

Hot stuff!

Steer clear of hot tubs, saunas, and steam rooms. Anything that raises your body temperature above 102°F (39°C) can harm your baby, particularly in the early weeks of pregnancy. If you have a fever, soak in a cool bath or take a tepid shower. Aspirin is best avoided. There is a question mark over its potential to cause birth defects; it interferes with blood clotting, which may increase the risk of excessive bleeding and blood flow problems in your baby.

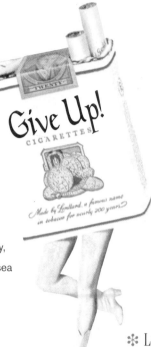

Smoking NIX NICOTINE!

Puffing while pregnant retards the growth of the fetus and placenta, which increases the risk of miscarriage, premature delivery, stillbirth, and sudden infant death syndrome (SIDS). The pregnant woman who smokes reduces her baby's brain power, is 60 percent more likely to have a child with a hare lip or cleft palate, and leaves herself open to a lot of dirty looks and disapproving comments. Giving it up is never easy, but pregnancy probably provides your best shot at sticking it out. Nausea can make smoking less enjoyable, and you have an important added incentive. There's also a lot of support available from various health information centers (*see* Useful Contacts, *pages 216–219*).

✳ Ladies! Give cigarettes their marching orders!

Alcohol and caffeine

An occasional sip is unlikely to harm your baby, but hitting the bottle can cause fetal alcohol syndrome (FAS), a bunch of abnormalities and behavioral problems that you don't want your baby to collect. The problem is that no one knows how much is safe—genetics play a part (and make black women more vulnerable) and binge drinking ups the ante. Most doctors advise going on the wagon, and pregnancy hormones often help out by making any alcohol taste foul. But don't panic if your sanity depends on a very occasional spritzer or glass of wine with a meal—a study of 400,000 American women found not a single case of FAS among women who had no more than 8.5 drinks a week. To be on the safe side, limit your intake to a maximum of one glass a week, and stick to standard measures—12 fluid ounces of beer, 5 fluid ounces of wine. Although the risks aren't as clearcut, you could also cut down on coffee, tea, and caffeine in general. Your tolerance for caffeine has probably taken a nosedive anyway, and too much can cause dehydration and might increase the risk of miscarriage.

KEEPING FLUID

Drink plenty of water. Aim for about six to eight glasses (4¼ pints/2 liters) a day. You'll want to pee all the time anyway, so you might as well make the trips to the bathroom worthwhile! Fluid intake is crucial at the moment. You are the pool lady in charge of filling up the customized flotation tank that is Junior's amniotic sac, and you've got to increase your blood production by 50 percent to make sure there's enough pumping through the placenta.

Some more baddies

Known no-nos include supplements and foods, such as liver and pâté, which contain high levels of retinol—the animal form of vitamin A. Your mom may dispute this (and, if she's like mine, probably will), saying she was told to eat liver during pregnancy because it's full of iron. It is, but intensive farming practices mean that nowadays liver is also full of retinol, and high doses have been linked to birth defects. It's not the only food that's changed. Some of the larger species of fish, such as shark, swordfish, tilefish, tuna, and king mackerel now contain high levels of PCBs (polychlorinated biphenols) and mercury and should be avoided—canned tuna from a reputable source is OK in moderation. Mercury is also given off during dental work involving amalgam fillings, although existing fillings are unlikely to cause problems.

Other stuff that can cause problems include the gases used in anesthetics, X-rays, and other sources of radiation (microwave ovens are OK), hot tubs, and lead—which gets you out of a lot of home-improvement jobs because this can be released when you strip old lead-based paint. Listeriosis, an infection that causes miscarriage, can be spread by raw or undercooked eggs and meat, and unpasteurized milk and soft cheeses that are made from it (such as brie and camembert). Raw or undercooked meat is also associated with toxoplasmosis, so wash your hands and work surfaces thoroughly after handling raw meat. Cats also carry toxoplasmosis, but there's no need to banish feline friends if you've had them for a long time, you've probably developed an immunity—ask your doctor for an antibody test.

If this is all news to you, and you're already a few weeks pregnant, don't panic. Your mother may not care to admit it, but in her day Martinis and Marlboros were the staple diet of millions of women who produced healthy babies. In an ideal world we'd all go on a health kick months before we start making babies, but in the real world more babies have been conceived after nights of drunken whoopee than over weekends of detox and dandelion tea.

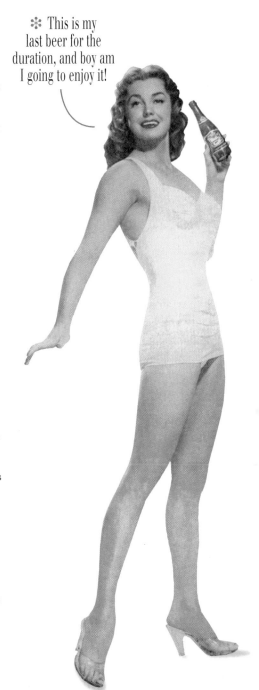

✳ This is my last beer for the duration, and boy am I going to enjoy it!

HOWDY PARTNER!

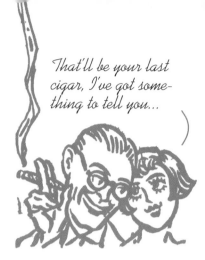

That'll be your last cigar, I've got something to tell you...

Prepare yourself for some eye-opening surprises from your partner as he acclimatizes to the idea of impending parenthood, and don't be shocked if he starts to sound more Neanderthal than New Man. Sure, he hasn't got the excuse of hormones, but it's important to remember that parenthood can be a pretty scary concept for guys, too.

Great news, sugar! Just let me out of this tux and I'll start boiling the water.

The huge social shifts that have taken place over the past 50 years or so mean that, in many ways, the script for your man's part is still at the rewrite stage. He's probably worked out that he won't be simply pacing corridors and handing out celebratory cigars, but he could be pretty hazy on what it is that he should do. Although he might not want to admit it, he's probably terrified at the prospect of actually being there on the big day. As a general rule, dads today want to be a lot more active in the process than their own fathers were, but role models are few and far between.

Let's face it girls, we sometimes send out mixed messages, particularly in the early stages, when pregnancy hormones start to surge. One day we'll insist on him sharing our pregnancy (whatever that means), and the next we'll complain that he hasn't got a clue what we're going through.

Talking time

Friends and family don't always help, either. While you're being bombarded with questions about morning sickness and delivery dates, he's probably fielding stuff like "Gee, what do you think a new baby will do to your golf handicap?"; and, "Does this mean you won't have time to use your Yankees season tickets?" Cultural differences can also come into play. It's only natural that your own upbringing will have had a strong influence on your approach to parenthood, so if you and your partner had different childhood experiences, it's a good idea to start swapping notes. Don't make any assumptions about childrearing. Parenthood is a bit like playing *Sim City*: it can turn leftwing liberals into authoritarian dictators, and strict disciplinarians into dribbling fools who can say nothing more articulate than "Coochy-coo!"

Some pretty strange thoughts can flit through a guy's gray matter when he discovers he's going to be a dad. You won't be far wrong if you accept that your boy is amazed, confused, delighted, excited, fascinated… all the way down to zonked. The same fears that have crossed your mind will occur to him, too: Will the baby be OK? Is it a boy? Is it a girl? Can we have sex? Will sex hurt the baby? What if I faint in the delivery room?

Fatherhood fears

Then comes the realization that he is now officially an adult, with very grown-up responsibilities. Right now, you probably have two incomes to support two people, but soon you'll be stretching one income to provide for three. He might have a few fears that won't even have occurred to you. You know that you are the baby's mother, but is he so certain of his status? Some psychologists claim that as many as one in three American men wonders whether he is really the father of his baby-to-be. The scientific literature is strangely silent on this point, but it's our guess that American men are no more suspicious, and no more cheated on, than other men around the world—it's just that they are encouraged to be upfront about their feelings, and the technology for establishing their status is so widely available.

Now is the time to take a serious look at your relationship. If there are any hairline faults, pregnancy and parenthood will soon split them open wider than the Grand Canyon. Minor irritations are magnified by a lack of sleep, and your ability to agree on the perfect dinner menu doesn't mean that you'll have the same approach to childcare. Now is the time to talk about everything from breast-feeding to who's going to be left holding the baby.

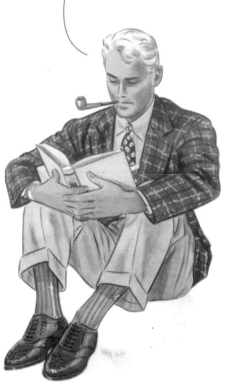

✳ Roger quickly mastered the fetal position while enjoying his last smoke.

FINANCIAL TIMES COUNTING THE COST

Most of the worries that consume expectant fathers focus on how they will cope financially and physically, and how the impending arrival will impact on their relationship. The only certainty is that there will be an impact, but you don't have to share Nora Ephron's gloomy view of parenthood ("A baby is a hand grenade thrown into a marriage"), and there's a lot to be said for the advice of columnist Elinor Goulding Smith: "The important thing is to keep your wits about you and borrow some money."

Great christening, darling — and there was enough in the collection plate to buy his first football.

Bean counters who seem to have nothing better to do than come up with new ways of terrifying parents-to-be have calculated that it costs a middle-income family around $150,000 to raise a child from birth to their 18th birthday. Add to that the cost of a college education and you'll need to find around $400,000. This is not the sort of loose change you're likely to find down the back of the couch. Had you sat down with this information and thought long and hard about it, you might never have got started on this baby business in the first place. Fortunately, accidents do happen, some people are cockeyed optimists, and babies get born—they have their own definition of the bottom line.

Even so, money's got to be mentioned. It's quite likely that, at least in the short term, you'll be making the switch from two incomes for two people to one income for three. Unless you're planning a bit of grand larceny, start getting used to the idea that you've said goodbye to disposable income and hello to disposable diapers.

Take stock of your finances and draw up a budget of your regular outgoings. A lot of these, like eating out and tickets to the movies, are going to change once baby makes three, but it's only when you know exactly what you're spending that you'll have any hope of taking control. Any savings that you can make now will be twice as valuable, because it will get you into the habit of budgeting and it can add up to a useful emergency fund. Skim through all those supplements in the weekend

✳ Judy bet the farm on Kentucky Derby Day — now she can afford a brand new baby.

TAX BREAKS

It pays to check out any applicable tax breaks—any extra cash will come in handy. In the United States, there are four that might apply: the Dependent Care Tax Credit, the Child Tax Credit, the Earned Income Tax Credit, and the Dependent Care Assistance Program.

papers that give tips on the best interest rates for savings or credit cards. Make a serious effort to whittle down any credit card, charge card, and store card balances, and take advantage of any interest-free periods. Set your priorities in terms of interest rates, paying off the cards with the highest charges first. It may also be worth taking out a personal loan to consolidate and clear any debts in one hit.

Housing is the biggest outlay for most of us, whether it's in the form of rent or mortgage payments. The first question to ask is: Will we have to move? And if so, when? Babies don't need a huge amount of space, although their equipment seems to. Pregnancy might conjure up pictures of pastel-painted nurseries, but there's no rule that says your baby needs a separate room. In fact, in some cultures, mothers are encouraged to keep their babies in the parental bedroom for the first year. The downside of this is that when the baby wakes up and cries, both mom and dad are woken up too, and two sleep-deprived parents is not good.

Make a list of any assets (and we're not talking great legs or a winning smile) that you can cash in if things get tight, and make a will. You need to think about who would raise your baby, and how it would be provided for. If both parents die without a will, any decisions about the baby's future will be in the hands of the state.

Then there's all the deeply depressing stuff such as life insurance. Right now, life insurance may sound like yet another unwanted expense, but it does provide priceless peace of mind. Policies don't have to be hugely expensive, particularly if you've become a non-smoker, and there are some that will provide a handy lump payment (which could cover college fees) if you go the distance. Don't make the mistake of thinking a stay-at-home mom doesn't need coverage. It would cost a fortune to employ a housekeeper, cook, cab driver, nurse, nanny, and teacher.

Hey guys, there's great womb service on Earth!

Alien INVASION!

Why are so many pregnancy books filled with soft-focus photos of calm women gazing wistfully out of windows, or serenely contemplating the years of bliss that lie ahead? For us, it was more a matter of gazing into the toilet, the strong paper bag, or whatever else we happened to be heaving into at the time, and cursing the spin doctor who came up with the term "morning sickness."

A few women are lucky enough to get minimal nausea in the morning, but it's much more common to have a puking peak in the morning followed by low-level nausea for the rest of the day. Blame it on hormones. In fact, for the next nine months, you can blame everything on hormones: tiredness, mood swings, insatiable sex drive, loss of libido, forgetfulness, cravings. There will be a huge array of changes, all triggered by the cocktail of body chemicals that is starting to slosh around your bloodstream.

Invasion of the body snatchers

Once your little embryo is embedded safely, it loses no time showing you who's boss. Many women complain to us that they feel they are nothing more than vessels and feeding stations. That's about the size of it, and you might as well get used to this right now. Don't be too tough on yourself if you sometimes feel that you have been taken over by aliens: in a way, you have been. Your

✳ I can't think why some pregnant women feel invaded by aliens.

✳ Nor me, honey—what's wrong with bug eyes anyway?

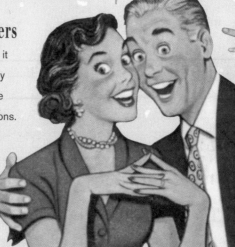

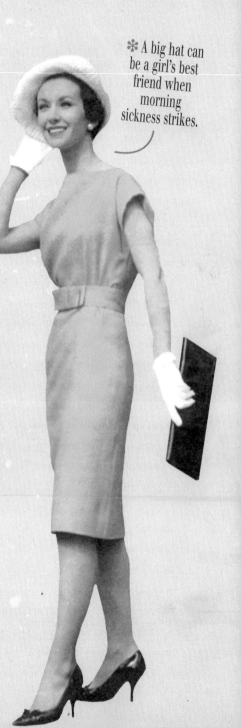

✳ A big hat can be a girl's best friend when morning sickness strikes.

own little space invader is formed of "alien" cells that are made up of a combination of genes from you and your partner. Normally the human body can get pretty snooty about cells that don't belong, and any suspicious strangers are seen off by the immune system, which is where pregnancy hormones come in. They are designed to head off any unpleasantness and override a lot of your normal body responses, such as menstrual bleeding, to create the perfect environment for a fetus.

Getting all hormonal

Hormones are going to play a big part in your life in the next few months, so you might as well find out more about these chemical cuties. You're probably already familiar with the two big ones: estrogen and progesterone. Throughout a woman's reproductive life, the ovaries produce progesterone and estrogen—there are actually several different types, but it's easier to lump them together as estrogen. Estrogen levels reach a peak around ovulation to ensure that the lining of the womb is all plush and cozy, ready to receive a fertilized egg, and progesterone rises after ovulation. If nothing happens, the levels fall off and the rich uterine lining is lost in a menstrual bleed. When conception occurs, levels of progesterone and estrogen remain high, and levels of HCG (human chorionic gonadtrophin, *see page 11*) rise, adding another ingredient to the chemical cocktail. This combination produces the hangover that is morning (hah!) sickness.

HCG is a messenger in more ways than one. Its primary role is to tell the ovaries to keep pumping out estrogen and progesterone, which are needed to put a stop to periods and ovulation for the rest of the pregnancy. Levels of HCG surge in the early stages of pregnancy, peaking between weeks seven and ten. As the placenta develops, it takes over and begins to produce the required estrogen and progesterone. When this happens, HCG levels fall off. Estrogen stimulates the growth of uterine muscle, and makes the womb strong enough to support your baby. It also activates breast changes, making nipples larger and prompting the development of milk glands. Progesterone relaxes uterine muscles, and damps down any contractions that could lead to miscarriage. These relaxant qualities also extend to your intestines, bowels, bladder, and arteries. This means that all your internal bits will be flexible enough to be squeezed out of the way by your expanding uterus. It also provides a further explanation for your constant need to pee, as sphincter control becomes a lost art. Other less-than-lovely side effects of all this progesterone include an increase in body temperature, and dizziness, because blood vessels become more dilated and blood pressure drops.

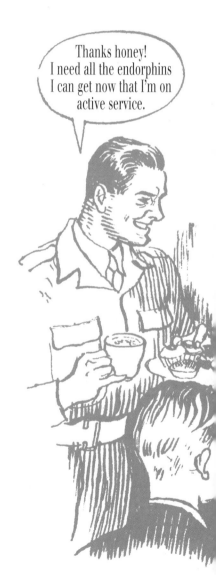

Thanks honey! I need all the endorphins I can get now that I'm on active service.

Relaxin is the Mr. Cool of body chemicals. It makes all your muscles and ligaments hang loose so that your pelvis can expand enough to let your baby out. The downside is that relaxin doesn't just soften pelvic ligaments: it gets to them all, which increases the risk of minor muscle injuries and backache.

Oxytocin is the clincher. It is responsible for all those contractions: the Braxton-Hicks practice ones as well as the eyepoppers of actual labor. If your baby is overdue, or things need speeding up, delivery can be induced with oxytocin in a drip. After delivery of the placenta, a shot of the hormone is often given to help contract the uterus.

At some stage, a thin dark line will appear down your tummy. Despite appearances, it's not a cut-along-the-dotted-line guide to a C-section. It's called the linea nigra, and it's caused by melanocyte stimulating hormone (MSH). It makes your nipples darker, and may cause an outbreak of blotchy patches on your forehead, nose, and cheeks. Women with pale skin get dark marks, while women with dark skin get paler marks. This is called chloasma, and there's not a lot you can do other than cover it with makeup and avoid the sun—and it will fade away after Junior arrives. MSH will also make around two-thirds of white women and one-third of black women get blotchy red dishpan hands, even if they have a dishwasher. Sunshine increases all these pigmentation changes, so when it's bright, be sure to wear an SPF 15 sunscreen or a hat. There's also some evidence that a shortage of folic acid intensifies the effect, so check that you're getting enough. This whacky effect on pigmentation also means it's a good idea to avoid bronzing sessions in the sun during pregnancy.

Anyone for endorphins?

Forget diamonds, endorphins are a girl's best friend. They're happy hormones that work in much the same way as morphine, and they take some of the *aaaarghh* out of labor pains. Endorphins are released throughout the pregnancy, which is why there will be times when you look a mess but feel utterly invincible. The bad news is that, like progesterone and estrogens, endorphins nosedive once your baby is born. Some medics believe that this is what causes the "baby blues," which so many women get around day three or four as a new mom.

It's active service that got you here in the first place!

For God's sake, take a cupcake, Joe. She's hormonal and she's got an icing gun!

As levels of HCG begin to subside, other hormones increase: human placental lactogen (HPL), insulin-like growth factors, and prolactin. This is the one that gives formerly flatchested women the cleavage they might have always craved, and turns everyday mammaries into the breasts of a goddess. Apart from making your man's day, HPL gets things ready for milk production. Toward the middle of the pregnancy it often leads to the secretion of small amounts of colostrum, a practice milk rich in protein (*see page 45*). This primes the pumping system and acts as an insurance policy in case Junior arrives early. Other hormones that increase during pregnancy include adrenaline and noradrenaline, which we'll talk about when we get to mood swings (*see pages 40–41*), and cortisone, which is why some allergic conditions clear up during pregnancy.

WHAT'S HAPPENING WHEN

FROM PEAS TO WATERMELONS

If the pregnancy hormones aren't already giving you nightmares, some of the comparisons made by pregnancy books when they talk about the stages of fetal development should do the trick nicely: "Your baby would now fit neatly into a walnut shell," and "She's about the same size and weight as an orange." If you read enough of them, you'll start to think that you're giving birth to the entire fresh produce aisle of a grocery store. However, we're not going to mess with tradition, so here's our fruity rundown of the changes to expect through the nine months.

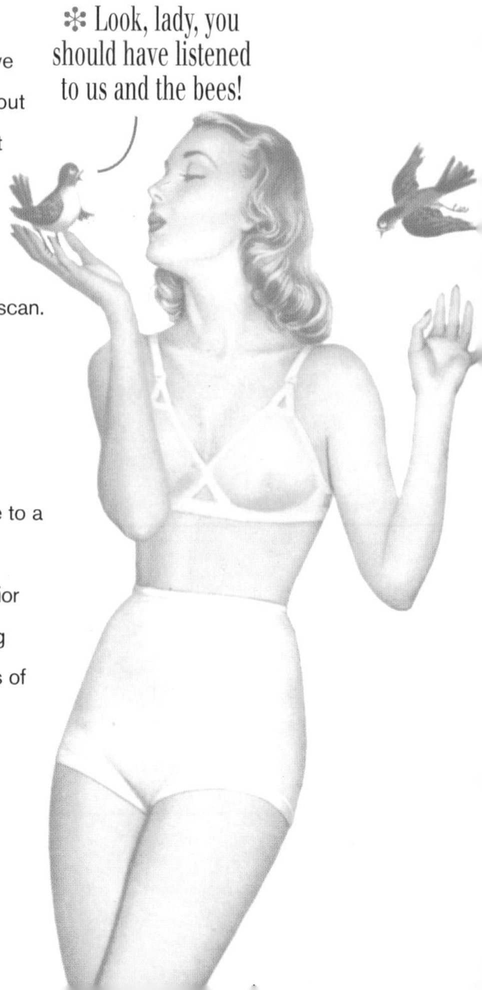
❊ Look, lady, you should have listened to us and the bees!

As mentioned earlier, when it comes to working out dates, the sums have about the same accuracy as calorie counts on the day that a diet goes out of the window. Officially, pregnancy begins from the first day of your last period, when you couldn't possibly be pregnant. Conception will actually have happened about three weeks later, but we'll stick to the official timetable and start our countdown from Week Six, when Junior could make his or her first appearance as a bit of a blip on an ultrasound scan.

Six weeks

Your baby is about the size of a pea, and would fit into a peanut shell with plenty of room to spare. It is recognizable as an embryo—it looks a bit like a lumpy tadpole squashed onto a stalk—but it bears very little resemblance to a human being, not even one who's really unphotogenic (there are several makeovers to go before Junior can pass for a person). Around this time, Junior will morph from what looks like a tadpole into a fish, and then into something with a stumpy tail that looks a bit like a monkey. By this time, basic versions of all the major organs are in place, but apart from the heart (which is already beating) they're not doing a lot. This is one of the most rapid periods of growth throughout the entire pregnancy, which is why it's also the period when your baby is most vulnerable to no-nos like alcohol and drugs.

GETTING BIGGER...
Eight weeks

At this stage, baby has grown to the size of a fava bean, a small strawberry, or a big olive, depending on your tastebuds. Speaking of buds, little ones have popped out and are turning into arms and legs—two of each, hopefully. By now, your baby is starting to look like a baby, rather than something from the tar pit in a B-movie. It is 10,000 times bigger than the single cell that set the wheels in motion, and expanding faster than a multinational in a virgin market.

Ten weeks

Now your baby is passing major milestones. The kidneys are now mature enough to produce their first pee, and—like many more to come—it's headed in your direction. Oh, and because it's growing bones (in the upper arms to begin with), it's now officially a fetus rather than an embryo. Baby is about 1 inch (2.5 cm) long and weighs ¼ ounce (10 g), about the same as a grape, and your womb is the size of an orange. Anyone for fruit salad? The stumpy arms and legs have frayed at the edges to make fingers and toes. These are perfect for sucking, which starts any day now. Junior's tail has disappeared, but there's no guarantee that you won't end up with a cheeky monkey a year or two down the line.

12 weeks

Your baby looks even more like a baby now, but its head is about the same size as its body, so it could also pass for a baby alien. The facial features can be clearly seen: a cute little snub nose, a large forehead (complete with wrinkles), and a definite chin. Ears and other protruberant bits will show up on an ultrasound scan, and your baby now has enough muscle and nervous system to start doing coordinated movements. In fruit terms, Junior is about the size of a plum.

RUBELLA

Rubella, or German measles, is the most dangerous infection that you can contract during pregnancy. At any other time it's little more than a bad cold, but in a fetus it can cause brain damage, deafness, heart defects, and intestinal abnormalities. If you didn't check your status before conceiving, it's one of the first tests your doctor will run (*see page 69*). If you don't have immunity, minimize your contact with young children.

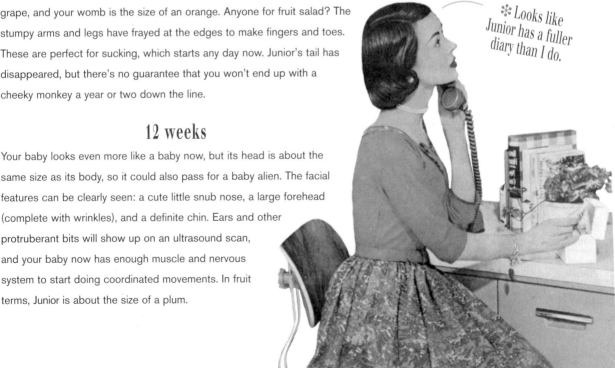

❋ Looks like Junior has a fuller diary than I do.

14 weeks

By now, your baby has a little groove under its nose, and the roof of the mouth has joined up. The first baby poop—ghastly, sticky, black stuff called meconium—starts to build up in the gut. Meconium looks more like tar than anything else, and if nobody warns you about it before baby takes his first poop, you will be convinced that your offspring had been conceived as the result of an alien abduction. By now, Junior is heading toward grapefruit status, weighing about 4 ounces (110 g) and measuring nearly 5 inches (12 cm).

Second trimester

By the fourth month, we start to see finishing touches like fingernails. The lungs start to do their share by pumping amniotic fluid, and wombside workouts contribute to the development of manual skills. You won't feel these at first, but sometime around the end of the fourth month or beginning of the fifth you'll start to notice a funny fluttery feeling, as if you really do have butterflies in your tummy. Soon after that, you'll notice definite movements—like kicks in the kidneys and an elbow in the ribs. Next time around, you tend to notice these movements earlier in the pregnancy— probably because you know what they are. Junior starts putting together a wardrobe: unfortunately, it consists solely of bum fluff called lanugo and a greasy white coating called vernix. Your baby now weighs around 5 ounces (150 g) and is about 6 inches (15 cm) long.

By month five, Junior weighs about 10 ounces (300 g) and is 10 inches (25 cm) long. He or she might already be developing irritating habits, like hiccupping or doing somersaults while you're trying to sleep. There's no hard evidence to confirm it, but we have found that the old wives' tales are actually right on this one: girls seem to get more hiccups than boys. The sense of hearing is well developed, and the baby might jump at sudden noises. The eyelids are still shut tight, but your baby will be

Tiniest tot

The smallest surviving baby ever born weighed just 10 ounces (283 g). Marian Chapman was born six weeks prematurely in England in 1938 (when there were no high-tech neonatal intensive care units and very low survival rates). The doctor who delivered her took an approach that would horrify most modern-day pediatricians—he used a fountain-pen filler to feed her brandy, glucose, and water once every hour for the first 30 hours of her life.

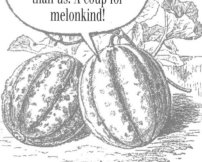

Apparently, Marlon, full-term human babies are just a bit smaller than us. A coup for melonkind!

aware of light, which reaches the womb as a rosy pink glow, and they may even turn away to avoid bright sunlight.

By month six, your baby is about the size of a cantaloupe, and weighs just over 1 pound (600 g). Finishing touches like eyebrows and lashes are thrown together, and the gray matter begins to flash signals around the brain, triggering scraps of memory. Be warned: unless you turn down the volume at the beginning and end of your favorite TV shows, you could find yourself using the theme tune of *Sex and the City* as a lullaby. Should your baby decide to arrive at around 25 weeks, he or she may have a 50 percent chance of survival and will be dependent on an NICU (neonatal intensive care unit).

Third trimester AND BIGGER!

You're on the home stretch now. Although the baby's growing faster than a credit card balance during the New Year sales, there's not much else going on. From now on, it's all about consolidation, and laying down supplies of brown fat—a special type of baby fat that acts as an internal heating system—and other healthy stuff, like iron. Most babies are around 4¼ pounds (1.9 kg) by the seven month mark, and space is running out fast. Early arrivals stand a good chance, although the lungs and liver are still lagging behind.

By month eight, Junior has piled on enough fat to pump out the wrinkles better than a Botox treatment. Your baby is now about the size of a small watermelon, weighing about 5½ pounds (2.5 kg) and is 17 inches (45 cm) long. By the delivery date, the average baby is around 7 pounds, 6 ounces (3.2 kg) but anything between 5½ pounds (2.5 kg) and 9 pounds, 5 ounces (4.2 kg) is thought to be OK. Personally, we'd say anything over 9 pounds is definitely not OK if you're the one who has to push it out (or you're the baby being squeezed out).

BIG IS BEAUTIFUL

When it comes to babies, small ain't beautiful. A baby who weighs less than 5½ pounds (2.5 kg) at birth is classified as having a low birthweight—bad news because it means they're more likely to run into health problems. Low birthweight babies are more likely to suffer neurological damage, respiratory infections, learning disorders, and behavioral problems. And as adults, they're at increased risk of heart disease.

✴ Don't get nervous—I wasn't this big when I came out!

IT MAKES ME SICK WHEN...

As we've already explained, the term "morning sickness" is deeply misleading. However, everyone uses this term, so we will, too—with apologies to those still barfing at bedtime. It's all a matter of degrees. Some women feel just a trifle unwell; others throw up once or twice; some are sick every day; and a few unlucky mothers-to-be are so badly sick that it goes by the name "hyperemesis gravidarum." If this happens, and constant vomiting leads to dehydration and weight loss, you will need specialized care.

✳ I like to keep my emergency crackers hidden in my compact.

The scandal of thalidomide—the morning sickness drug that caused fetal deformities—has made doctors cautious about prescribing medicines to stop nausea. But if you've got it bad, there are certain anti-nausea drugs, which dull the part of your brain that tells your tummy it's time to throw up. If all else fails, you might get to look like an *ER* extra, and be hooked up to a drip to restore your nutrient and fluid balance.

Double is trouble

It may not feel like it right now, but morning sickness is actually a good sign because it means that there's a plentiful supply of the hormones needed to maintain your pregnancy. That's why women who are carrying twins tend to get it worse: they have an extra helping of hormones. There are old wives' tales that suggest that one sex or the other is more likely to make you sick. These vary depending on which old wife is telling the tale, and in which part of the world it's being told.

In most cases, morning sickness starts to subside sometime after the 12th week of pregnancy, and completely fades away by the 16th week. However, if it stops suddenly, or abates much earlier in the pregnancy, it might mean that there is a problem with your hormone levels. A sudden drop in hormone levels is associated with miscarriage.

HEADY STUFF!

Snack time

One reason for nausea being at its worst in the mornings is that it is associated with low blood sugar, or hypoglycemia. When you're asleep, you're not eating (unless you have developed a truly special talent), so blood sugar levels are at their lowest when you wake up. This can also trigger other symptoms, such as lightheadedness, lack of energy, and shaking. Hormone levels and blood sugar levels are clearly linked, but the science is still at the early stages, and scientists aren't sure which is the chicken and which is the egg, as it were. A number of studies have shown that women with bad PMS may be more sensitive to blood sugar fluctuations, or experience a sharp drop in their levels a few days before each period. This also explains why chocolate and candy become utterly irresistible at certain times of the month.

Sugar, sugar

We don't know whether it is hormones that play havoc with blood sugar levels, or a lack of blood sugar that affects hormones levels—either way, it makes you feel lousy. This explains why so many helpful home remedies for sickness involve snacking or sugary drinks: they provide a quick shot of blood sugar. Because of their relatively simple chemical structure, sugary drinks, candies, and refined carbohydrates such as white bread and crackers, are quickly converted into blood sugars. There may be times (such as first thing in the morning) when you need the quick fix that these foods provide. However, in the long run it's much healthier to eat complex carbohydrates such as whole-grain breads and cereals. It takes longer to convert complex carbohydrates into blood sugars, so they provide a constant dripfeed of blood sugar. By contrast, simple carbohydrates and

GINGER MAGIC

Ginger is a well-known remedy for relief of morning sickness.

Make a ginger infusion by adding two teaspoons of grated or chopped gingerroot to 1 cup of boiling water. Leave it to infuse for five minutes.

To make candied ginger, peel a large piece of fresh ginger and chop it into small cubes. In a pan, dissolve 1 cup of sugar in 4 cups of water to make a syrup. Then add the chopped ginger and simmer until the root has softened. Leave in the syrup overnight and then pack in airtight containers.

Don't look unless you're at least three months gone!

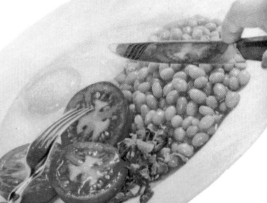

sugary foods flood quickly into the bloodstream, and your body pumps out large amounts of insulin to convert them into energy or fat stores. This stabilizes sugar levels, and you can start to crave something sweet again. Sugary foods may also see you piling on unwanted pounds without getting much in the way of nutrients.

A simple way to avoid these sugar highs and lows is to eat light meals and frequent snacks, which are probably much more appealing anyway. The easiest things to keep down are often salads and simple light meals, like broiled chicken or fish with steamed vegetables. Foods that are most likely to make you throw up include those that are highly spiced, deep-fried, or covered in thick, creamy sauces. It's largely a case of suck it and see—a friend of mine swears by a protein snack at bedtime and a carbohydrate snack in the morning, preferably before getting out of bed. If you can persuade someone to bring it in on a tray along with the morning paper, so much the better.

I may be eating for two, but I'm still the queen of portion control.

Food and other fixes

In the real world you cannot just lie on the chaise lounge all day, so you will need to find some strategies to help minimize morning sickness. Carry combat rations at all times. Tried and tested morning sickness remedies include dry crackers, nuts, dried fruit, sweet cookies, rice cakes, bananas, and apples. It's also worth trying candied ginger, ginger chewing gum, and anything else containing ginger, because it's a natural stomach settler and has been used in China for centuries to treat digestive problems. Make your own ginger infusion (*see box on page 37*) and add some honey or lemon to taste. Even if you don't normally like ginger, give it a try—you might be surprised. One friend of mine who loathed ginger and was a complete caffeine junkie before pregnancy

❋ I'm off to the den—the smell of my tobacco and beer, and the sight of my sweater, are making my wife nauseous.

found herself drinking gallons of the stuff. Flat Coke or Pepsi and ginger ale also work for some women, although this doesn't fit with all that doctorly advice about cutting down on caffeine and sugar. Freezer pops made with children's oral rehydration formula are also very palatable for sufferers of nausea.

Another simple remedy for nausea from Asia is acupressure. It works along the same lines as acupuncture, but uses pressure instead of needles, which makes it a lot more convenient and means you can do it to yourself. There's a point in the middle of your wrist that is said to control nausea; it's three fingerwidths from the point at which your hand joins your wrist. If you're righthanded, the right wrist will probably be the most effective; lefthanders should press on the left wrist. A simpler solution is to buy a pair of acupressure bands. You'll probably find them in the motion sickness section at drugstores.

Some natural therapists recommend taking extra vitamin B6 to relieve morning sickness. The anecdotal evidence is promising, but there's no solid science to prove that it works. So long as you don't exceed the recommended dietary intake (1.6 milligrams), it won't do any harm.

Certain smells can trigger gut-churning nausea—particularly nasty ones like tobacco and stale sweat—which can be a nightmare if you work with a chain-smoker who has only a passing acquaintance with soap. Trust me, barfing over a boss with BO is not a good career move. Deep breathing, a blast of fresh air, or sniffing a piece of ginger or a cut lemon may help to avert an employment crisis.

The two most important things to remember about morning sickness are that it won't last, and that you should replace any fluids and nutrients as soon as you think they will stay down.

MOOD SWINGS AND ROUNDABOUTS

t's a gear shift any Formula One team would kill for: you can switch from überbabe to crybaby in under ten seconds. One minute you're daydreaming about pushing a stroller through the park, the birds are singing, and everything's rosy. The next you're daydreaming about pushing your partner over a cliff, the TV's too loud, and you're feeling so blue you could burst into tears.

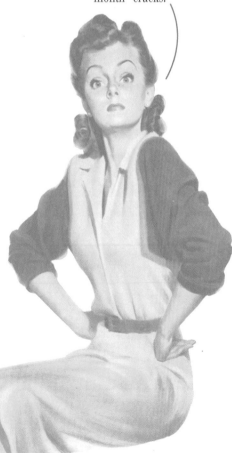

❊ Well, at least you can stop with the "time-of-the-month" cracks!

It may feel as if you're going crazy, but mood swings come with the territory, particularly in the early weeks when your body and soul are struggling to come to terms with a deluge of hormones and unanswered questions.

That H word again

The symptoms are similar to a bad case of PMS, and many of the same hormones are to blame. Round up all the usual suspects, like progesterone and estrogens, and throw in some adrenaline and noradrenaline. Your heart beats faster, you breathe more rapidly, you can't eat, and your hands and feet are sweaty. No, you're not in love: it's the adrenaline cranking up your metabolic rate by 25 percent. This pumps more oxygen-rich blood to the embryo to get rid of extra carbon dioxide waste as fast as possible, and to train the cardiovascular system for the extra load it has to carry. The hormones also provide an extra shot of energy, although it might not feel like it now.

Adrenaline and noradrenaline are the "on" switches for the fight-or-flight response. In the days when we all lived in split-level caves and it was politically correct to wear fur, these hormones gave us an evolutionary edge. The fight-or-flight response was meant to be a quick fix, a swift shot of chemicals to deal with a short-term threat. These days, we don't have to do battle with dinner, and if we remain on alert we become edgy, nervous, and even nauseous. These symptoms are all associated with long-term stress— and the early stages of pregnancy. Levels of adrenaline and noradrenaline rise steadily during pregnancy, and this can tip our emotions into overload.

What mood swings? I'm just doing this to make my legs grow longer.

If hormones aren't enough to send you over the edge, the worries and questions of pregnancy probably will be. Are you ready for this?—Probably not, no one really is. Will your baby be OK?—Almost certainly, the odds are stacked firmly in your favor. How will you cope with the labor?—However feels right at the time. How will you juggle parenthood and a job?—You don't even know yet whether you'll want to, but try talking to people with young children to see how they keep the balls in the air. Will your body ever return to normal?—It depends on your definition of normal, and how much work and time you're prepared to put in. What if you lose the baby?—Miscarriage is a tragedy, but most often occurs in the early weeks, and is often nature's way of saying that there's something seriously wrong.

Blues mothers HAVE A GOOD CRY!

If you hadn't planned on becoming pregnant, you might have very mixed feelings about the prospect of parenthood, and lots of practical problems to overcome. There's no rule that says you have to be overjoyed at the news, so don't be afraid to admit that you're afraid. It's perfectly normal, and it doesn't mean you will love your baby any less. Although baby blues and postpartum depression (these *are* different) are widely acknowledged and openly discussed, recent research suggests that depression is often more severe during pregnancy than after it. Everything gets blamed on the hormones, but there may be other reasons to feel desperate. Perhaps the timing isn't terrific, or it's going to be tough financially. It's scary being a single parent, but if you're not in a stable relationship, or your man decides he's not ready to be a dad, you may have no choice in the matter. The world doesn't stop just because you're pregnant. Serious illness, unemployment, and accidents still happen, and can have an impact on you and your baby. Stress is a part of life and there's no avoiding it, not even in the womb.

BEAT THE BLUES

Recognize the signs of stress: sweaty palms, a thumping heart, muscle tension, wide eyes, and nostrils flaring like a racehorse that's just finished the Derby. Find a release that works. We don't recommend practicing primal scream therapy on the boss, but gentle exercise, a massage, meditation, or a good heart-to-heart with a friend will all help.

FEARS AND FATIGUE

Pagan priestess or pudding? Self-esteem and your body image shape your attitude to pregnancy. Some women revel in the physical affirmation of their own fertility, and see swelling breasts and a round belly as symbols of strength and beauty. Others view their vanishing waistline with dismay. Women who have struggled with an eating disorder are particularly vulnerable at this time, and are likely to need a sympathetic ear or a little extra support (*see* Useful Contacts, *pages 216–219,* for groups that can help).

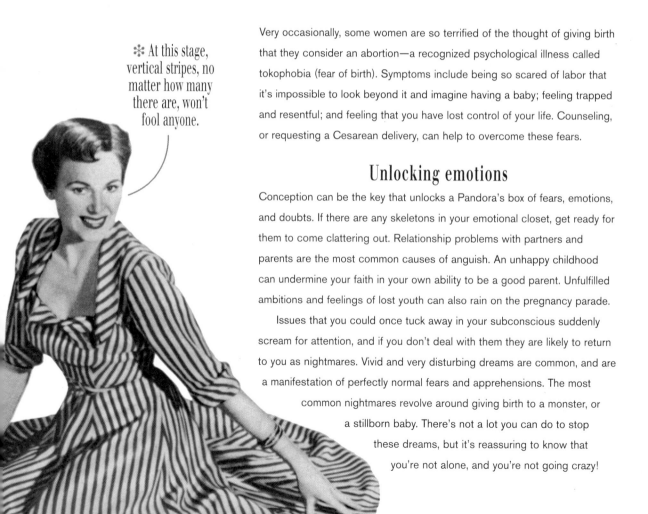

❊ At this stage, vertical stripes, no matter how many there are, won't fool anyone.

Very occasionally, some women are so terrified of the thought of giving birth that they consider an abortion—a recognized psychological illness called tokophobia (fear of birth). Symptoms include being so scared of labor that it's impossible to look beyond it and imagine having a baby; feeling trapped and resentful; and feeling that you have lost control of your life. Counseling, or requesting a Cesarean delivery, can help to overcome these fears.

Unlocking emotions

Conception can be the key that unlocks a Pandora's box of fears, emotions, and doubts. If there are any skeletons in your emotional closet, get ready for them to come clattering out. Relationship problems with partners and parents are the most common causes of anguish. An unhappy childhood can undermine your faith in your own ability to be a good parent. Unfulfilled ambitions and feelings of lost youth can also rain on the pregnancy parade.

Issues that you could once tuck away in your subconscious suddenly scream for attention, and if you don't deal with them they are likely to return to you as nightmares. Vivid and very disturbing dreams are common, and are a manifestation of perfectly normal fears and apprehensions. The most common nightmares revolve around giving birth to a monster, or a stillborn baby. There's not a lot you can do to stop these dreams, but it's reassuring to know that you're not alone, and you're not going crazy!

YAWN!

Naps, sleep, and utter exhaustion

Tiredness is something that you probably won't really have experienced until you're pregnant. You might have thought you were tired after running a marathon, or after staying up all night studying for a big exam, but that was a little light lethargy compared with the all-encompassing, utter, and total exhaustion that comes in the early stages of pregnancy.

You'll suddenly find yourself longing for lunchtime naps, falling asleep on the couch at seven o'clock, or turning down dinner invitations because you know you'll never make it past the appetizer. You probably don't have a hint of a bump, but your baby has taken control. Carry an alarm clock and catnap when you can. Many offices have medical rooms with beds. If you fancy the fresh air, find a park bench, but leave your purse at work. If you're in a car pool, take a back seat and nap on the journey. On public transport, ask a friendly face to wake you at your stop and watch your belongings.

This fatigue makes a bit more sense when you realize that, by the 12th week of pregnancy, your fetus is tiny but perfectly formed, and growing at a phenomenal rate. There is so much happening down there, it's no wonder you need to lie down. Physical factors that contribute to fatigue include: the increased metabolic rate that makes your body work overtime; high levels of progesterone that make you drowsy; possible anemia; and disturbed sleep patterns (all that getting up during the night to pee).

Don't fight it. This is one battle you can't win, and you shouldn't try to. Give in gracefully and get as much sleep as possible. You're going to need it. Make sure you're eating well; ask your doctor if you need an iron supplement; employ a cleaner, or ask your partner to do more around the house; confide in a work friend who might be able to lighten the load; take the easy option whenever it's presented; catnap when you can; if you have children, ask friends and family to take them for the day, and go to bed.

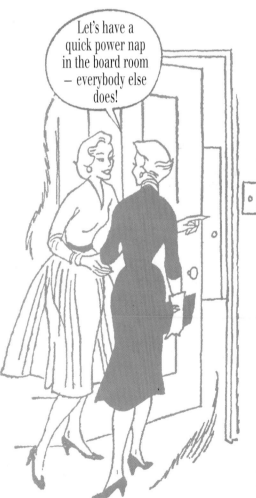

Let's have a quick power nap in the board room — everybody else does!

THANKS FOR THE MAMMARIES

AND OTHER DEVELOPMENTS

Your cup will start to runneth over very early in pregnancy. Breast changes occur as early as the third or fourth week, when some women experience an itchy, prickly, tingling sensation, particularly around the nipple. This is caused by increased blood flow, and may continue for some weeks. While it does, you may be overcome with the sudden urge to slip into the washroom for a good scratch, or let the shop assistant at Victoria's Secret in on your secret.

By Week Six of the pregnancy, there's enough estrogen and progesterone racing around your system to stimulate the development of the ducts and glands needed for milk production. Your hooters will start to holler for attention, particularly if you tend to experience breast tenderness just before periods. If you are in denial and haven't done a pregnancy test by the eighth week, some other thin blue lines will probably announce the news: tiny bluish veins will emerge all over your breasts.

Each breast is made up of lobes that contain little bunches of alveoli—these contain cells that produce and propel milk along the ducts (*see diagram opposite*). You're born with a certain number of these alveoli and ducts, and they expand during pregnancy. You also grow new ones, which means that your pre-pregnancy breast size has nothing to do with your breast-feeding ability. Many formerly flatchested women squirt milk quite happily, while Pamela Anderson lookalikes (without added silicone) can struggle to maintain their supply. Speaking of silicone, it shouldn't get in the way of your ability to breast-feed, but breast reduction surgery might.

The nipples and areolae (the pigmented areas surrounding the nipples) become larger and darker as the pregnancy progresses, particularly if you have a dark complexion. This may be an all over gradual transformation, or a bit hit-and-miss and blotchy. In the later

ESSENTIALS

BREAST FACTS

Each breast lobe contains alveoli, which contain inner milk-producing cells and outer myo-epithelial cells to propel milk toward the milk ducts. The milk collects in the ampullae (reservoirs) behind the nipple.

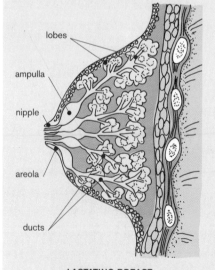

lobes
ampulla
nipple
areola
ducts

LACTATING BREAST

stages, patches of pigmentation might form secondary circles around the areolae. Around Week Ten, little bumps, known as Montgomery's tubercles, on the areolae become more prominent. Their primary purpose is to pump out sebum to lubricate the skin and keep the nipples soft and supple. If you're breast-feeding, you'll want your tubercles to be giving it the full Monty!

Around Week 16, you'll start producing colostrum, a runny practice milk that's packed with protein and antibodies, and you might want to express a drop or two out of curiosity, or to prime the plumbing. It won't do any harm, and in some cultures it's encouraged. Using your whole hand, gently squeeze from the outer breast toward the nipple. Alternatively, gently squeeze the breast at the areola and pull the tip of the nipple out slightly. Some men find this incredibly erotic, so don't be shocked if your man wants to lend a hand.

Minor irritations

All sorts of strange little things start to happen when you're pregnant, some of which your mother or physician might forget to mention: Ptyalism, for instance—isn't that a word to whet the appetite for learning? As for what it means, it's excessive salivation, often just before you throw up or get heartburn. It starts around Week Eight. Heartburn can appear early on, but tends to be most troublesome in the last ten weeks or so, when progesterone relaxes the valve that prevents gastric acid from entering the esophagus, and your bulging belly is pushing everything else northward. We'll put the heat on heartburn later on (*see page 150*).

Your sense of smell is heightened, and may become so sensitive that it hurts. You will experience previously attractive aromas as assaults on the olfactory system. Some say this hyperdeveloped sense of smell is a primitive survival mechanism that prevents pregnant women from eating rancid foods, which might pose a threat to the baby. These days we've got refrigeration, so evolution should give us a break.

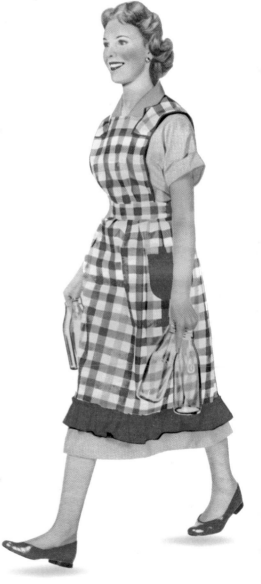

❋ Gerda wondered how on earth she was going to fill so many milk bottles.

GIMME, GIMME, GIMME!

Once, you dreamed of Prada and Armani. Now, you'd kill for pretzels and apple pie, with extra ice cream and tomato ketchup on the side—and maybe a pickle for good measure. Cravings come with the territory and some scientists say they're positive, because they could be the body's way of saying that it needs an important nutrient. This isn't as silly as it might sound.

✻ I keep my fruit on my head so that no one else can get at it.

Early in pregnancy, a lot of women tend to go weak at the knees over citrus fruit, and can easily polish off a pound, or three, of oranges or grapefruit. This is one time when greed is great, because citrus fruit is bursting with folate and vitamin C, both important for a healthy baby and pregnancy. Another common craving, which tends to kick in a little later on in pregnancy, is for red meat. You may find yourself sitting down to a steak supper several times a week, and even vegetarians have been known to hover around the meat counter looking longingly—and very guiltily—at slabs of prime rib. Again, it adds up: red meat provides a rich and readily accessible source of iron, and as the pregnancy advances, you need more and more of this to boost hemoglobin levels, which supply you and your baby with much-needed oxygen.

If you are a vegetarian or vegan and are starting to get strong cravings for meat, listen to your body rather than your conscience, because it could be trying to tell you something really important. Ask your doctor for a blood test to make sure that you're not anemic and take an iron supplement if you are—vegetarian versions, such as Floradix, are available in most health stores. A good tip for boosting iron levels is to drink orange juice with iron-rich foods because vitamin C enhances iron absorption. It's also a good idea to keep a food journal to double-check that you're getting all the B-group vitamins and protein you need—plant sources don't provide the same comprehensive range of meat and animal products, so it's important to eat a mix of legumes and grains (and take your prenatal vitamins!).

IRON BOOSTERS

Iron tablets taste unspeakably awful and often cause constipation. Avoid them by boosting your intake of iron-rich foods. Good sources include red meat and organ meats (but avoid liver), green leafy vegetables, eggs, seaweed, wheat germ, and dried fruit. Drink orange juice with iron-rich foods because vitamin C boosts absorption by a factor of four.

CRAVING CONTROL
Oh for an Oreo

There is just one catch with this primitive programming theory. These instincts were honed long before chocolate sundaes, Oreos, and family-size pizzas. We scream for ice cream, but our body could just be looking for calcium. Once we would have wandered into the woods to pick fruit and nuts, but now we can wander down the confectionery aisle and pick up jumbo packs of fruit-and-nut chocolate.

You can't ignore your cravings, but you can try to control them—substitute frozen yogurt for ice cream, for instance—and make sure that your baby's nutritional needs come first. Be extra vigilant if your cravings focus on foods and snacks that contain a lot of sugar, salt, sodium, or hydrogenated fats (also known as trans fats). Sugary foods are loaded with calories and very little else. They'll add to your waistline measurement, but will provide few of the nutrients you need to grow a baby. Salty foods can cause fluid retention (and you really don't want to look or feel more bloated than you already are!). Hydrogenated fats are bad news for your heart, and tend to hang out in unhealthy processed foods that you should be cutting down on anyway.

Occasionally, cravings focus on items that aren't even foods, such as soil, coal, ice, or chalk. This is called pica, and no one really knows what causes it, although the usual suspects (yep, those hormones again) are a safe bet. Another theory is that pica is triggered by iron deficiency, so it's worth asking your doctor to check you aren't low. Heaven knows why, but some women also find that the charcoal tablets sold in drugstores will help—and at least you know where they've been. Fight these strange cravings if you can, but if you do find yourself baking soil in the oven in an attempt to sterilize it for supper, you won't be the first. I must stress that this is not a recommendation, but it's probably marginally safer than simply eating the garden *au naturel*.

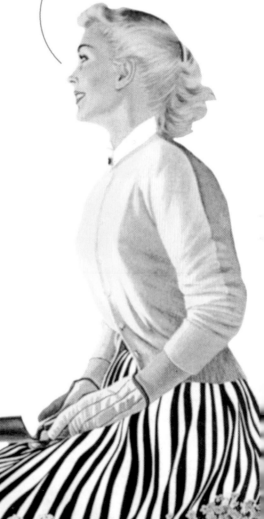

✳ When I get the munchies, I need some real Mississippi Mud Pie.

OLD WIVES' WISDOM?

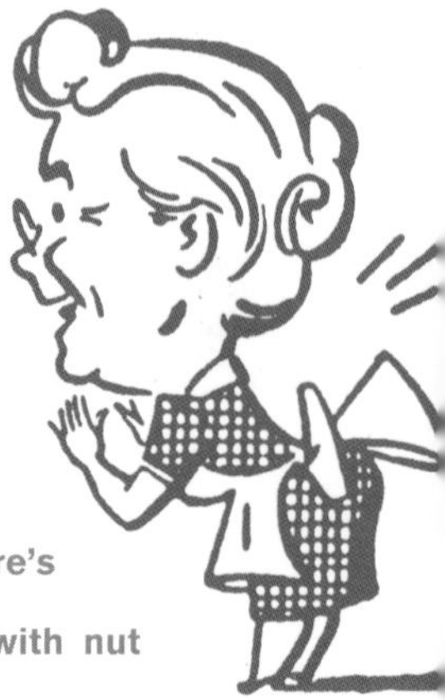

Don't go listenin' to any other old wives' tales but mine!

All sorts of silly stories have grown up around cravings and other aspects of pregnancy. There's absolutely no truth in the tale that eating too many strawberries will give your child a strawberry birthmark. Nor is it true that when your baby is older, he or she will like the foods you craved in pregnancy—in fact, if anything, it may work the other way around. If you eat a lot of peanuts during pregnancy, there's a risk that your baby will develop an allergy, because the protein associated with nut allergies can cross the placenta.

�֎ Relax, my dear; it's a scientific fact that earwax consistency is a reliable gender predictor.

�֎ Oh really? And who told you that? Your mother or her mother?

In a lot of countries around the Mediterranean, they say that babies will be born with a birthmark if a pregnant woman is denied whatever it is that she wants—I'll have a George Clooney with a bit of vintage Paul Newman on the side, please. These stories have absolutely no basis in fact, but what a great way of motivating your partner to scour the neighborhood for all-night access to Hershey bars, gefilte fish, or whatever it is that happens to be busting your tastebuds.

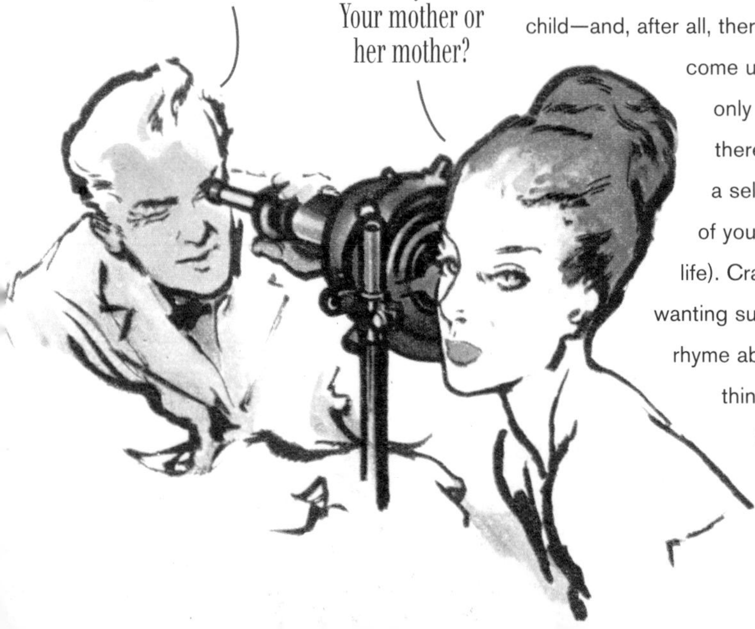

Some old wives' tales are supposed to reveal the gender of your child—and, after all, there is a 50–50 chance that these techniques will come up with the right answer. Personally, I suspect the only thing that they reveal is how many whacky people there are out there. However, for what it's worth, here's a selection. Eat a clove of garlic: if the smell seeps out of your pores you will have a boy (and sink your social life). Craving the crusts of bread means that it's a boy; wanting sugar signifies a girl (and may explain that nursery rhyme about girls being made of sugar and spice and all things nice). Pee in a jar with a large spoonful of Drain-o in it: if it turns green, it's a girl; if it goes blue, it's a boy. If you're graceful, it's a girl; if you're tripping over your feet, it's a boy (the only snag with this one is that we all get clumsy when our bump makes our feet disappear from view). Pull down your lower lid and look at the white of your eye: if you see a vein that's V-shaped or branches, you're having a girl (or maybe it just means you need a good night's sleep). If someone asks to see your hands and you show them palms up, it's a girl; palms down, it's a boy.

Suspending a wedding ring over your hand or belly to see if it makes a circular motion or goes straight up and down is supposed to show the gender of your child, but the problem is that 50 percent of old wives say a circle signifies a girl and the other half say it signifies a boy. The same applies to all the stories about carrying high or low, up front, or around your sides. There's only one thing your bump can really tell you: you're pregnant. You've worked that one out already.

Then there are the stories about starting labor—having sex (possibly, because orgasm releases hormones that might start the action); a good belly laugh (no, but a laugh's always welcome); a curry or very spicy food (it may activate your bowels but is unlikely to wake up your womb); foot rubs (why on earth would they?); and playing with your nipples, or having someone else do it for you (there is actually some truth in this one because it releases the right hormones).

The nipple story is not the only old wives' tale to have a grain of truth. Take the one about losing a tooth for every pregnancy: statistically, there is actually a link between having children and losing teeth. For a while, people thought this might have something to do with calcium loss, but a recent study came up with a new theory—stress. Researchers found that new moms are just as good at brushing and flossing, but increased stress levels mean that their gums are more sensitive to the bacteria which do all the damage. The fact that pregnancy hormones also make gums softer and more likely to bleed probably doesn't help either.

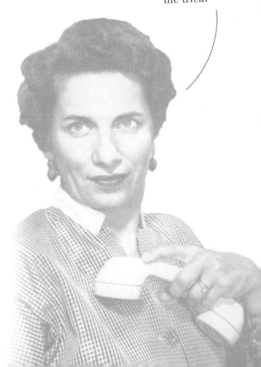

✻ It's a boy! Didn't I tell you that wearing blue panties would do the trick?

Pregnancy, your partner,

Time to trade up to a bigger four-legged friend; my moseyin' days are over.

and the rest of the world

Once you've applied to join the parenthood club, a series of subtle shifts in attitude and interests will begin. Dog-eared family photos will take on a new meaning: "Oh my God, will you look at the nose on her!" You may find yourself catching up with friends and family who have young children, picturing your life a year or two down the line, and wondering what on earth you're getting yourself into.

❋ As fatherhood loomed, Herb put on an impressive display of upper arm strength.

Mothers, mothers-in-law, and other close female relations can provide a wealth of information and support, while the men can give your guy a few tips about his new supporting role. Try to keep everyone near, but not too close for comfort. It's not always easy, and in some families it might seem impossible, but a united front and a few ground rules will go a long way.

They heard it on the grapevine

When it comes to breaking the news, it's the grapevine—and who hears what, and when—that really matters. Some people delight in keeping a secret, while others will spread the word quicker than a computer virus attacking an email address book. In the scheme of things, this is a pretty minor issue, but it's worth thinking about who needs to know, when they need to know, and how you are going to tell them.

Some parents-to-be can't wait to tell the world, and some don't have any choice. Severe morning sickness, or friends who are quick to guess, can blow the secret. Many couples prefer to get through the early weeks, when there is a higher risk of miscarriage, before letting on. Older mothers who have an increased risk of having a Down's syndrome baby may want to know the results of a CVS or amnio first (*see pages 84–87*), particularly if any family or friends are opposed to abortion, and are unlikely to accept a decision to terminate the pregnancy. However, when you do delay breaking the news, people can feel hurt, or worried why you didn't trust them. It's a balancing act, but it's your balancing act. Even if you do temporarily lose your footing with a family member or friend, any disappointment should soon be forgotten. If it's not, try to take a pragmatic view. If someone creates problems this early in the game, do you really want them around when things start getting sticky?

Make mine a double — or a triple

Where once your partner's credit card bill or his team's injury list sent shivers down his spine, now the sight of triplets might throw him into a tailspin. You can point out that natural triplets are very rare. Nowadays, two out of three sets of triplets are because of fertility treatments. Only nonidentical twins run in families, and even then, only on the woman's side. The odds of having identical twins are the same for everyone: around one in 250. If you're a nonidentical (fraternal) twin, you're five times more likely to have fraternal twins than a mother who isn't. It's also more likely to happen if you're over 30, when the ovaries are more likely to launch eggs in pairs to compensate for declining fertility. The odds of having nonidentical twins can also vary between different ethnic groups. With gonadoptrophin injections or IVF therapy, there is a 20–40 percent chance of multiple pregnancies.

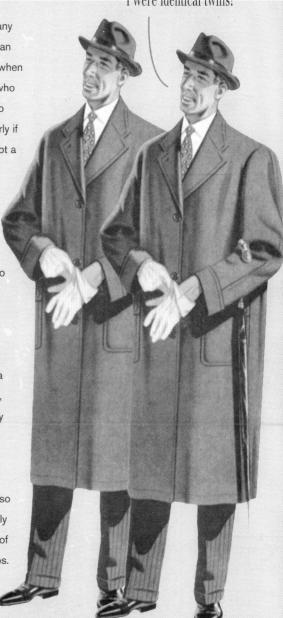

✳ Gee, honey, didn't you realize that Chandler and I were identical twins?

MISCARRIAGE AND OTHER WORRIES

Worrying about miscarriage, or serious problems with the baby, is the most common reason for keeping quiet in the early weeks. Miscarriage (or spontaneous abortion, which is the term doctors tend to use) can happen any time up to the 24th week of pregnancy. If anything goes wrong after this, the baby is said to be stillborn. Thankfully, late miscarriage is rare. Most miscarriages happen in the early weeks, often before the pregnancy is even known about.

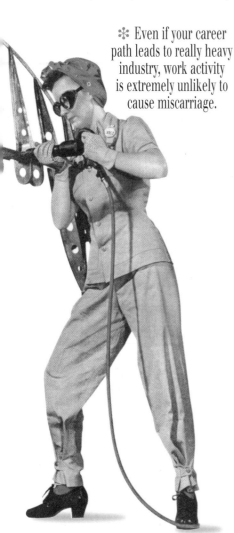

✳ Even if your career path leads to really heavy industry, work activity is extremely unlikely to cause miscarriage.

Around 25–30 percent of confirmed pregnancies end in miscarriage, but some estimates put the real incidence at two in every five pregnancies (this is often age-related because the older the mother, the higher the risk of miscarriage). These figures sound frightening, so it's worth remembering that miscarriage usually happens for a reason, most often because there is something so seriously wrong with the fetus that it cannot survive. There's also a huge difference, both emotionally and physically, between miscarrying a very early pregnancy before it is well established and later losses.

Causes of miscarriage

Most miscarriages occur in the first 12 weeks, and 70 percent of these are caused by chromosomal abnormalities or diseases of the fertilized egg. An egg's failure to stick firmly to the womb, and problems with the trophoblast (which becomes the placenta), account for most of the others. Causes include: chronic health problems, such as renal disease or hypertension; a very high fever; exposure to radiation; and exposure to some drugs. Risk factors include age (it's most likely to happen if you are under 16 and over 35), and unhealthy habits such as smoking, excessive drinking, and drug abuse. Drinking four or more cups of coffee a day might also increase the risk.

It's probably more helpful to be reassured about things that don't cause miscarriage. No one can guarantee that computers are absolutely safe, but there's no credible evidence that they increase the chances of losing a baby. The same goes for microwaves, so long as there's nothing wrong with the door seal. Sex isn't a problem, unless your doctor advises against it. A minor trip or fall shouldn't do any harm either, although a Scarlett O'Hara on the stairs might. Unless your physician has warned you to take it easy, it should be quite safe to lift moderately heavy weights such as shopping bags or toddlers, but make sure you use good back safety methods—always bend at the knees and keep a straight back.

Later loss

The most common cause of late miscarriage is an "incompetent" cervix, which means that the cervix is a bit slack, lousy at timekeeping, and opens up too early. Some women are born with this condition, or it can be the result of some sort of trauma, or your mother taking a synthetic estrogen called diethylstilbestrol (DES) when she was pregnant with you. It is a relatively uncommon problem, but it is on the increase because of the success of cervical screening programs. Such programs have saved thousands of lives by providing early warnings of cancer, but they have also caused a big increase in the number of women having multiple cervical procedures such as cone biopsies, which can potentially weaken the cervix. There are also other uterine abnormalities that can be associated with an incompetent cervix, such as a bicornate or heart-shaped uterus.

This form of incompetence doesn't respond to pep talks, but there is a simple solution: a cervical cerclage. It's a circular running stitch, a bit like the drawstring in a purse, and it keeps the cervix shut. It's usually done late in the first trimester under a regional or perhaps a spinal anesthetic once scans and prenatal tests confirm that the fetus is fine. It should be taken out a week or two before the due date, so if you have one and things start to happen ahead of schedule, make sure that you get to a hospital pronto—medical staff should treat this as a matter of urgency.

PCOS

The right drugs and lifestyle can improve the outlook if you have polycystic ovary syndrome, aka PCOS. Polycystic ovaries interfere with normal ovulation and may also increase the risk of miscarriage. They are generally benign, but they often go hand-in-hand with a package of hormonal imbalances affecting fertility across the board, from conception to completion. The right drugs and weight loss can sometimes improve the outlook. (*See* Useful Contacts, *pages 216–219,* for more information.)

Signs of trouble

Sometimes there is no sign of trouble until a routine scan shows that the fetus is no longer alive. However, some mothers instinctively sense that something is wrong, so if you are worried, trust your instincts and ask your nurse-midwife or doctor for a check. A good provider won't mind false alarms and will be more than happy to put your mind at ease.

Bleeding can be bad news, and it must be checked out. However, it doesn't always mean that you will lose your baby—50 percent of women who experience threatened miscarriage in the first trimester go on to have healthy babies. It's also not unusual to get a bit of spotting around the time of your first or second missed period. The later any bleeding occurs, and the heavier it is, the more cause there is for concern, as it might be a sign that the placenta is separating from the uterine wall. A brownish-red discharge is less ominous than a bright red discharge. Never use a tampon if you bleed during pregnancy, and bring any used pads when you visit your physician. This sounds gross, but it will give your doctor an idea of the amount of blood loss.

❉ Never suffer in silence if you think there is something wrong; the medical team is there to help you, not discuss the weather.

What happens next?

If you suspect something's wrong, there is no point chewing your fingernails and fearing the worst—seek medical attention. A physical examination, blood tests, and ultrasound will reveal whether there really is a problem, and what to do if there is. Tests carried out at this time can provide useful clues to what went wrong, and help to prevent it happening again. Any miscarriage can be physically and

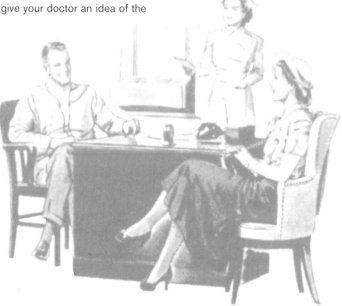

ESSENTIALS

ECTOPIC PREGNANCY

If you get severe abdominal pain in the early weeks, it could mean you have an ectopic pregnancy, in which the fertilized egg becomes stuck in a Fallopian tube instead of the womb (rarer locations are the ovary, cervix, or other places in the abdomen). This happens in one in 50 pregnancies, and is often caused by scarring in the tubes, caused by earlier pelvic infections. If the pregnancy is ectopic it's usually doomed, but with early intervention medical treatment may be possible. This will conserve the tube and increase the chances of a later successful pregnancy.

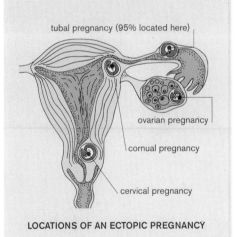

tubal pregnancy (95% located here)

ovarian pregnancy

cornual pregnancy

cervical pregnancy

LOCATIONS OF AN ECTOPIC PREGNANCY

emotionally traumatic, particularly if you have lost a baby before, it took a long time to get pregnant in the first place, or you had made it through the early, risky weeks. Even women who had mixed feelings about being pregnant can experience deep feelings of sadness. Give yourself time to grieve, and don't be afraid to ask for help or support. You might have a lot of questions, or you might just feel numb. Feelings of guilt are very common, but are usually absolutely groundless, so don't beat yourself up. Remember that you are probably not the only one who is hurting. Your partner has lost a potential child too, and he might find it harder to show how upset he is, or feel that he has to be strong for you. (*See* Useful Contacts, *pages 216–219*, for support groups.)

Recurrent miscarriage

If you've had one miscarriage (or more), the fear of another is never far from your mind. Statistically, the odds are in your favor, even if you've had more than one miscarriage. An incompetent cervix, as we've already mentioned, is one cause of recurrent miscarriage that can be treated. Other causes are related to conditions that can create clotting abnormalities and affect placental function, such as antiphospholipid syndrome. Basically, this means that you have antibodies that make your blood too sticky, and this interferes with the normal function of the placenta and causes pregnancy complications such as miscarriage, early pre-eclampsia, separation of the placenta, or even smaller babies. Once it's been diagnosed using a simple blood test, it can be treated. Other causes include chromosomal abnormalities in the parents or hormonal defects. Sometimes no cause is found and your doctor will monitor you closely during the next pregnancy.

ACTIONS AND REACTIONS

When you decide to start spreading the word about your pregnancy, it can be a good idea to draw up a list. Check it against your address book to avoid any embarrassing omissions. Pregnancy shrinks the brain with more certainty than a hot wash cycle for a silk blouse, and it can play havoc with your memory. Like so many things at the moment, it's all down to hormones. However, if your great aunt Gertie has escaped Alzheimer's and still has all her gray matter intact, she will feel upset at being left out.

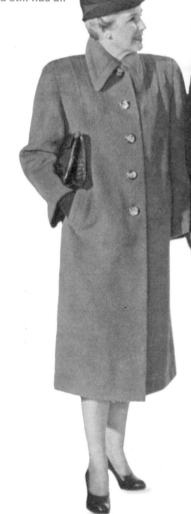

Then there's the thorny question of who to tell first. How would your mom feel if she discovered you'd told a girlfriend first? Would your mother-in-law ever forgive you if she found that your mom knew before she did? What do you do when one side of the family is old school and starchy, while the other is new age and hangs loose? You do what you should always do in pregnancy: whatever feels right for you. Let's face it, if people are going to get niggly over the announcement, what on earth will they be like when it comes to the really serious stuff, like names? Every family is different, and only you and your partner know how family members are likely to react.

Mixed emotions

One of the hardest things for some women is telling a close friend or family member who can't have children. Statistically, this scenario is quite common: one in six couples seeks medical advice about fertility at some time. Just as it's impossible to imagine the feelings that pregnancy unlocks, it's also impossible to imagine the heartache of wanting children but being unable to conceive, or the emotional rollercoaster and financial sacrifice of fertility treatment. However, you can make an effort to tell your friend or family member in a way that acknowledges his or her own situation. Of course, he or she will be delighted for you, but it's only natural that there will also be

✽ Oh Pa, you don't have to increase my allowance now that I'm pregnant! I own the company, remember?

sadness, envy, and anger. Break the news one-to-one in a private place, so that your friend can smash a few plates or have a good cry. Let him or her know that you understand the urge to break down in tears: given your hormone-crazed state, you might find yourself joining in. There's no point trying to hide any feelings of happiness and excitement, and it will look phony if you try. Take your cues from your friend. Some childless people want to share every moment of a friend's pregnancy, while others will run a mile to avoid it.

Mom's the word

One of the big pluses of pregnancy is that it might, perhaps, finally, just maybe, convince your mother that you're an adult. The government naively thinks that we come of age at 18, but mothers are never really convinced. You might have had the key to the door for years now, but as far as your mother is concerned, you're still her little girl and you've only ever been playing at "house." This finally changes when her own little girl announces that she's producing a little girl or boy of her own.

If it doesn't, and your mother (or, worse still, mother-in-law) starts trying to lay down the law—her law, that is—put your foot down, gently but very firmly. We know it's not easy, and nobody wants a showdown, but there's absolutely no point trying to avoid this one. The more you skirt around the issue, the greater the chance of a major bustup. It's your bump, it will be your baby, and the sooner everyone understands this, the better. You don't have to be rude. Try saying: "Thanks, but I think the advice has changed on that one," or "It's really very kind of you to offer, but we haven't made a decision on that yet." You won't go far wrong if you start with "Thank you" and slip in an all-important "but" afterward. Remember to say it with a smile. Another handy tactic is to slip in little questions that highlight how thinking has changed. "Is it true that they used

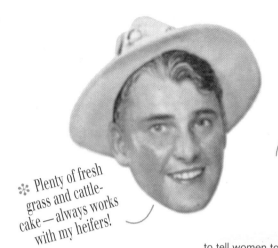

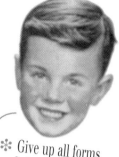

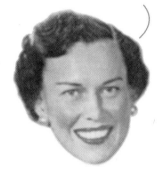

* Plenty of fresh grass and cattle-cake—always works with my heifers!

* Give up all forms of pleasure other than housework, now and forever!

* Now remember, dear, momma knows best!

to tell women to eat lots of liver? It's funny, now they say we shouldn't eat it at all." A lot has changed since our moms had us. Morning sickness is accepted as a real condition; bumps are beautiful and there to be flaunted; bottle-feeding isn't promoted in hospitals; and we know that putting a baby to sleep on his or her back reduces the risk of crib death.

Know nonsense

If you're stuck with a particularly irritating know-it-all, you could try dragging her—preferably not kicking and screaming—into the 21st century. Showing her a few carefully chosen websites and chatrooms might get the message across without causing too much fallout. Chatrooms are also a brilliant way of airing issues that are causing friction. If you can't find an online debate about your particular gripe, you can always cheat and start one. If your know-it-all is also a technophobe who thinks that the Internet is something to do with fishing, use the old standby of a "friend" with a problem: "So-and-so in my prenatal class is at her wit's end trying to fend off unwanted advice, but she's worried about upsetting her mom/mother-in-law/sister. What do you think she should do?"

Family members aren't unique in their capacity to drive you nuts: friends and coworkers can be just as pushy. When it comes to babies, everybody seems to have an opinion, and the chances are that you will hear every single one of them, no matter how crazy, contradictory, or confusing. Short of creating a wardrobe of T-shirts emblazoned with messages like "Yes, I

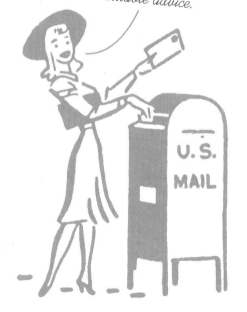

Bernice doesn't answer her phone— I guess I'll just have to mail her my invaluable advice.

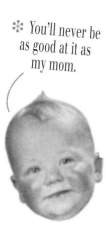

※ You'll never be
as good at it as
my mom.

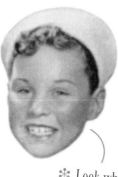

※ Look what
formula milk
did for me!

※ Eat up all your
crusts or your baby
won't have lovely
curly hair like mine!

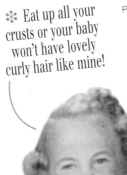

※ Your mother
says to tell you to
eat a pound
of liver a day.

do know," "No more advice, puhleeeease!" and "I don't want to hear it,"
there's not a lot you can do. If you really can't face another person telling
you what to do, try the old toddler-taming tactic: don't look, it only
encourages them. Refuse to make eye contact, and give short, dead end
answers if they persist.

New men, same old problem

Women tend to be the worst offenders when it comes to excess advice, but
men are not immune. One of the snags with SNAGs (sensitive new age
guys) is that because they're in touch with their caring, sharing side, they
feel free to chip in with advice. Back in your dad's day, no self-respecting
man who wasn't a doctor would admit to knowing a thing about pregnancy
and all that "messy business." Now, dads and dads-to-be can be among the
worst baby bores. It's not too bad when they stick to subjects they
understand, like the fear of fainting, but it's infuriating when they hold forth
on subjects such as labor pains. Many men will sanctimoniously insist that a
pregnant woman's body should be a temple, while treating their own like a
fast food joint on the other side of town. You can spot these guys in prenatal
classes. They will ask for extra homework, and come out with lines like: "We
want a drugfree delivery," and "We would never consider a C-section." As
one sister put it: "Honey, let me know when you can go to the john and
produce a watermelon. Then you'll be qualified to comment and may have
something worth listening to."

FAMILY TREE

Ask your mom and mom-in-law if
there is any history of hereditary
diseases, which could make it
important to know the sex of your
baby. Girls are X-rated, and every
egg we produce contains an X
chromosome. Boys have both X
and Y ratings. If an X sperm
meets the egg, you get a girl; if a
Y sperm gets there first, it's a boy.
Conditions such as hemophilia
and muscular dystrophy are X-
linked and more likely in boys
because they have only one copy
of the X chromosome.

BECOMING PUBLIC PROPERTY

A funny thing happens on the way to the maternity ward... Somewhere along the line, your personal space evaporates and you keep running into people who assume that you are deaf, or stupid, or both. This starts to happen when your bump begins to bulge and your pregnancy can no longer be mistaken for an extra burger or two, and reaches a climax by the time you're ready to drop. By this stage, you'll also be so sick of telling complete strangers when the baby's due that you may be tempted to print up business cards with all the relevant details. Like it or not, you are now public property.

> Honestly, Sybil, if I'd known how often people were going to pinch and poke, I'd have bought an armor-plated jacket like yours.

This is one of the few downsides of joining the club called parenthood—there are hundreds of thousands of long-standing members who can't wait to give the new girls a bit of friendly, or otherwise, advice. It's usually well meaning and there will be times that you will love the chance to chat about scans or crazy cravings. But there could be other times when you'll be left speechless—or perhaps not—with fury at people's rudeness.

Take coffee, for instance—a lot of pregnant women do. As mentioned earlier, there's some evidence that it may, repeat may, be linked with an increased risk of miscarriage, but the scare stories center on women who drink large doses! There's no suggestion that coffee—or tea—in moderation will do any harm at all. Many physicians advise their patients to cut back, but admit there's very little evidence of problems with a normal intake. Still, you may find someone sidling up to you in Starbucks and asking, "Are you sure you should be drinking that? Don't you know it may be harmful?" Sally, a nurse-midwife says, "I can't tell you how angry this made me feel. I used to get a double latte on my way into work and most days there'd be this woman by the door who'd tut and shake her head disapprovingly. Finally, she couldn't hold back any more and gave me this massive lecture on the damage I was supposedly doing to my baby. OK, she didn't know I was a nurse-midwife, but why on earth should she assume that I was some brainless breeding machine and that she knew it all? I'm not sure which got me mad the most, her rudeness or her ignorance. The next day I gave her copies of all the information I could find on caffeine in pregnancy—the facts, from medical journals and research papers, not the pseudo-science that's sometimes peddled by magazines and newspapers. I don't think she knew what hit her—but at least it wasn't my fist. I never did see her again, so maybe she realized how rude she'd been."

Pregnancy police BUTT OUT!

For a real explosion of public outrage, it's alcohol and cigarettes that are the most combustible combination. Smoking is undoubtedly dangerous for babies—whether they're unborn, newborn, or on their way to becoming grown-ups—but nicotine is also addictive and it can be incredibly difficult to give it up. Jessica, 41, says, "I hate the fact that I smoke and I've tried many times to give up, but I just can't seem to beat it. Before I got pregnant, I smoked 40 or 50 cigarettes a day, but as soon as I found out, I cut right back to five a day. I know that's not perfect, but it's a big improvement. If you haven't smoked, it's hard to understand—but that doesn't give people the right to be verbally abusive. One woman actually spat at me and called me a child killer; it was like something from the Jerry Springer show."

Attitudes may be hardening, according to Miriam, a vegetarian who also enjoys a glass of wine, or a beer, with meals. "I'm not saying I am a heavy drinker, but I enjoy an occasional glass of wine when eating out. During my most recent pregnancy, I was having a very, very weak white wine spritzer in a restaurant and did get a few comments—and quite frankly I told people where they could

SMOKE SIGNALS

Here are a few tricks that may help you quit smoking: Keep a journal to identify the times you most want a cigarette, and try to avoid them. Don't eat spicy foods (you probably aren't anyway) because they often trigger cravings. Fresh fruit, vegetables, and juice may take the edge off cravings. Chew sugar-free gum. Take a shower, or soak in a tub as often as you can. Every day you don't smoke put the money into a jar and buy yourself a treat when you've saved up enough.

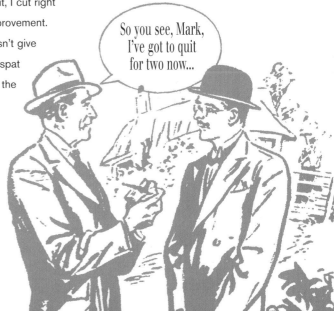

So you see, Mark, I've got to quit for two now...

file them. I don't eat meat and I think it's abhorrent to kill animals for food, but I would never dream of haranguing complete strangers in burger bars, so why do people think they have the right to tell me what to do? I wouldn't condone a woman getting really drunk during pregnancy, but I really don't see the problem with having a very occasional drink. Pregnant women have rights, too." Thresholds vary from person to person, so a few sips are probably OK, but always bear in mind that alcohol is a known teratogen and don't overdo it (*see page 22*).

✽ And this is for you, Goody Two Shoes—I always take my fruit juice in a beer glass.

Fending off unwanted advice

So what do you say when you're on the receiving end of this sort of unwanted advice—or abuse? A lot depends on who's delivering the lecture and how stressed you feel at the time, but you wouldn't be the first to suggest that someone take a long walk off a short pier. If it's someone whose opinion, or friendship, you value, talk to them. If smoking's the issue, explain how you're feeling and how difficult it is to quit. If you ask for their support, you'll probably defuse their condemnation. If it's a less clear-cut risk factor such as coffee, be upfront and say that you really don't believe moderate, with the emphasis on moderate, consumption is dangerous—and do they really think that you'd knowingly harm your own child? If the criticism is coming from someone you hardly know, you can try pointing out, ever so politely, that it's actually none of their business. Other suggestions include:

☞ "Oh, please, may I have your autograph? I've never met a perfect person before."

☞ "I always order a cocktail on the rocks—it's fun to see how many busybodies it will flush out of the woodwork. You're the first, but the night is still young." (Then point out that you've ordered a non-alcoholic cocktail.)

☞ "Now see what you've done! Your rudeness is making me so tense that I'll have to have another drink/cigarette/coffee... just to calm down."

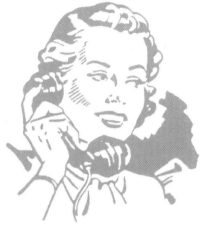

� It was the president on the line again, with yet another of his tips on prenatal nutrition.

☞ "Actually I'm not really pregnant, I'm a researcher and I'm doing a study about intolerance and stupidity in our society. Thanks so much for your contribution, it's been very helpful."

One of the really strange things about all this concern in the community is that it often vanishes the moment you set foot on a crowded train or bus. Suddenly all those people who were so worried about your health and safety, and that of your baby, are perfectly happy to hide behind newspapers or books and let you strap-hang, being bumped and jostled, for the whole ride home. OK, some men say in their defense that sexual equality has got them so confused that they don't dare offer a seat. Well, guys, most pregnant women will be more than delighted to accept, and usually with a smile and a thank you. One mom-in-the-making got so tired of standing during a long commute that she started saying, very loudly, "If there's a man on the bus who isn't pregnant, I'd really appreciate it if he'd offer me a seat."

Perhaps it's some primitive response to the visible proof of your fertility, or perhaps it's just an excuse for a grope, but all sorts of people will start patting your belly in a slightly proprietorial way. Some women enjoy this familiarity, and it can be lovely when the hands that are stroking your stomach are attached to a partner, a parent, or a friend. However, when it's the old man who packs your groceries at the store, or a stranger at the bus stop, it's hard not to become all Clint Eastwood and snarl, "Go ahead punk, make my day," before using your knee to inflict an injury that will add to the infertility statistics. Most people will get the hint when you flinch and try to maneuver your belly out of reach. If you encounter a serial stroker, try to explain, as nicely as you can, that you really don't enjoy being pawed.

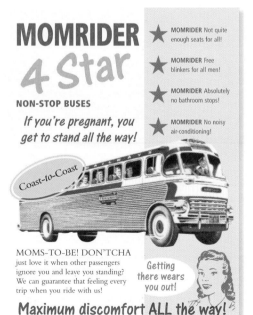

MOMRIDER 4 Star

NON-STOP BUSES

If you're pregnant, you get to stand all the way!

★ MOMRIDER Not quite enough seats for all!

★ MOMRIDER Free blinkers for all men!

★ MOMRIDER Absolutely no bathroom stops!

★ MOMRIDER No noisy air-conditioning!

Coast-to-Coast

MOMS-TO-BE! DON'TCHA just love it when other passengers ignore you and leave you standing? We can guarantee that feeling every trip when you ride with us!

Getting there wears you out!

Maximum discomfort ALL the way!

WORK IT OUT

I f you thought pregnancy had a funny effect on you, just wait until you break the news to your boss. Employers can react to staff pregnancies in the most astonishing ways. If you're lucky, you may be given a bunch of flowers and be told to take it easy, but don't hold your breath. Sadly, there are also employers who view staff pregnancies as an expensive and disruptive inconvenience, and can be so unpleasant they make Ebeneezer Scrooge look like a goodwill ambassador for the United Nations. There are a lot of variables, some of which will determine your rights and options.

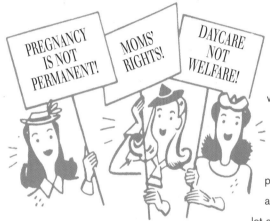

If you are employed, start investigating your rights to antenatal and maternity leave and whether or not you can return to work after the birth. Talk to coworkers who already have children; they'll be able to tell you whether your company goes by the book or offers a bit more flexibility. Your rights will vary depending on where you live, whom you work for, and how long you've been in your job. As a rough guide, companies with more than 15 employees have to give you time off—although many personnel offices view pregnancy as a disease and refer to maternity leave as a "period of disability." It's cockeyed, but it's useful to know because a lot of the employment laws that protect people with disability also cover pregnancy. Maternity leave usually allows a minimum of six weeks off (six to eight if you've had a C-section) and this can be paid, unpaid, or covered by a cocktail of sick pay, personal days, vacation, and disability insurance.

TAKE CARE

Once you've decided on the type of care—nursery, baby sitter, or nanny—start looking while you're still pregnant. Long waiting lists are not unusual and they're usually a very good sign—if lots of parents are clamoring for the same nursery or carer, it means they're doing something right.

Telling the boss

Find out where you stand before breaking the news to your boss—it puts you in a much better bargaining position. Work out what *you* want to do and put together a plan that could make it happen, but try to see things from your boss's side, too, and come up with answers to all the questions he or she is likely to ask. To avoid confusion and protect your back, keep your employer informed of everything in writing. There's no guarantee that your line manager or boss won't change, and if a new one isn't as sympathetic, you'll be in a much better position if any agreements are documented.

Decide when you want to leave, and when you plan to return—but try not to paint yourself into a corner; your view may change when your bump has become a baby. Doctors consider the 38th week of pregnancy a good time to leave work, but some women prefer to continue beyond this, and not everyone has a choice financially. Find out what the company offers in terms of support (if you're really lucky, there might be childcare facilities). Investigate jobsharing or part-time work for at least the first year after the birth. It may be possible to work some of your hours from home. Company handbooks, your union, and coworkers who already have kids are good sources of information. If you work for a company with 50 or more employees you're also covered by the 1993 Federal Family and Medical Leave Act, which guarantees your job, or one that's just as good, when you take up to 12 weeks off.

If you are self-employed, take a realistic look at your workload and consider offloading some or getting in extra help. Working from home may give you increased flexibility, but when there's all that breast-feeding and sleep deprivation to contend with, you may think otherwise. Many first-timers naively believe that it will be easy to fit the newborn into a high-powered working life; they think that they will leap effortlessly from the delivery table/birthing pool/Anasazi birthing stool and carry on as usual. After all, how hard can it be to look after something so tiny? Second-or-third-timers will have more realistic views of their own capacities, but should also remember that every pregnancy is different. Even if you slid through your first on velvet runners, the second might not be so easy.

❊ I wish Cindy was back from maternity leave—I have got no idea how to work this photocopier.

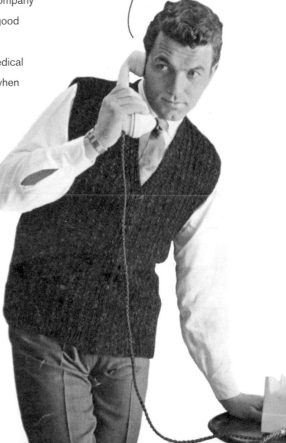

CARE OPTIONS

The first big question that you'll have to find an answer to is the type of care you'd like. OK, so you've already got a few ideas: kid-glove, four-star, platinum, maybe gold at a push (start getting used to that word; about nine months from now you'll probably be doing a lot of it.) When it comes to medical professionals, you have three basic options: an obstetrician, a family physician, or a certified midwife. But there are some other ideas that you may not have considered, like doulas—which is another way of going back to the basics of childbirth support and shows how attitudes can go full circle.

Doula is a Greek word for a woman servant and that's basically what they're all about. After a century of increasingly medicalized childbirth, a lot of women are going back to the idea that, when it comes to delivering babies, it's other women who are the most likely to offer practical help and support. Doulas don't have formal medical training and can't take the place of a physician or obstetrician, but they can work alongside medical professionals to provide a more personal touch. There's evidence that having a birth coach, such as a doula, speeds up the delivery because you're less likely to feel stressed and start pumping out the wrong hormones. They also ensure that there's a familiar face throughout the delivery—shift changes and medical emergencies mean that you may not always have the same nurse, or your own physician. If you are considering a doula, look for a birth coach who's certified by the Doulas of North America, *see* Useful Contacts, *pages 216–219.*

Qualified midwives offer the same sort of sisterly support, with the added advantage of medical training—look for the letters CM (certified midwife) or CNM (certified nurse-midwife) after their name, because in some states anyone can call themselves a midwife and a lay midwife is definitely not the same as a CM. Midwives take a more natural approach to childbirth and are qualified to handle low-risk pregnancies and straightforward deliveries.

✳ I love looking after the baby — it's this what-is-she-thinking frilly apron that I can't stand.

TO FP OR NOT FP
Doing it group or solo

Doctors who specialize in pregnancy, childbirth, and pediatrics are known as
family physicians (FP). They've had more training than a standard MD and
should be able to cope with most complications. If problems arise,
they could call in a specialist, such as an obstetrician, but it's the FP who
calls the shots. Some FPs are one-man—or one-woman—bands and run
solo practices with a back-up doctor to cover for times they're not available.
In theory, a solo practice means that you'll always have the same physician
and by the time that you go into labor you'll have developed a
comfortable trusting partnership—just like in the movies. But in
practice, and the real world, babies don't time their arrival with
their physician's work schedule in mind and no one, no matter
how caring and committed, can be available 24/7. Choosing a
group practice guarantees a familiar face, but you may like
some of the physicians more than others, and fate has a nasty
habit of delivering the dud—relatively speaking, that is.

Obstetricians are the heavy hitters, childbirth specialists
who are trained to handle any and every emergency—the real
ones, not the broken nail variety. If you're a high-risk mom-to-be,
or have a prepregnancy problem such as diabetes or hypertension,
go straight to the top and book yourself in with an obstetrician. For
superspecialized care if your problem is particularly complex, you may
be referred to a perinatologist.

Once you've decided on an obstetrician, FP, or midwife, how do you
find a good one? Ask friends and family who've had babies recently
for any recommendations, or warnings. Remember that style's
important, too (isn't it always!). Some may be more comfortable with an FP
who will take control and tell you what's going to happen. But if you'd
prefer more of a partnership, make sure your doctor sees it that way, too.

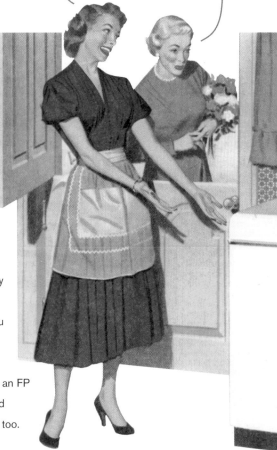

❊ And on
Mondays I get to
sit on my brand
new 1100 rpm
washing machine!

❊ Isn't that what
got you in this mess
in the first place?

Leg it, girls!

Tests, doctors, AND MORE TESTS

"**D**ear diary, what's wrong with me? I used to fill you up with fun things, like movies and lunches with the girls. Now the only dates I've got are with my doctor and midwife. I wouldn't mind so much if my doctor looked like Brad Pitt, but the only hope this guy has of getting my pulse racing is by telling me I'm having twins..." Congratulations: you've just enrolled in the bootee camp that is antenatal care.

✳ The only test I've ever done was for Mr. Hitchcock.

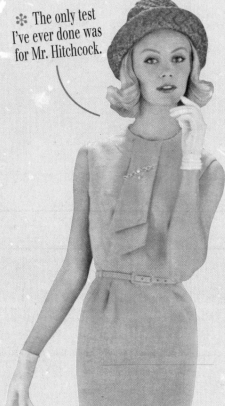

Don't be tempted to skip any of the tests scheduled during your pregnancy, even though they can be a drag—most of them are early warning systems for serious problems. Don't be afraid to ask questions, and make sure you understand what's being done and why. Think through the implications: What will you do if something does show up? If you wouldn't consider an abortion, you might say no to invasive tests for abnormalities. However, they may reveal such things as heart defects, which can be corrected with surgery, and at least they will help you to prepare for what lies ahead.

Truth and consequences

A nurse-midwife, doctor, or obstetrician will want to know your full gynecological history. This is not the time to be coy. Medical staff are there to care, not judge, so there's no need for embarrassment. The chances are they've probably seen and heard things that you can't even imagine. Your partner does not need to know everything that's happened in the past, but your doctor does. Everything you say is confidential, and it does not always have to appear in your notes. If it does, there's usually an abbreviation or Latin term that can be used if you are worried that your partner might see your records.

You are likely to be asked questions about your menstrual history and last period; if you've been pregnant before, and if so what happened; if you've ever had an abnormal Pap smear, and if so whether you had surgery; if there is a history of twins in your or your partner's family; and whether you were taking any medicines or recreational drugs at the time of conception.

Your first prenatal appointment is between Weeks 8 and 12, and could be with an obstetrician, family practitioner, nurse practitioner, or a nurse-midwife. It involves a few basic checks, including weight, blood pressure, and urine and blood analysis. These provide a baseline for later readings, and help your physician to assess the importance of any changes. What is "normal" will vary from woman to woman and throughout the pregnancy.

A small blood sample will be taken to check your blood group, rhesus and rubella status, and general health. It might also be tested for HIV. You might have an internal examination to assess the cervix and uterus, and a Pap smear to make sure that there are no precancerous abnormalities. You'll be weighed, so that the practitioner can track how much you gain, and don't be surprised if you are asked your shoe size: it's a good clue to the size of your pelvis. Anything above size 4½ indicates that there's enough room for your baby's head to get through. You should also be given advice on potential hazards and recommended diet.

The number of tests and appointments you have depends on: your age; your gynecological history; whether it's a multiple pregnancy; and whether you have any chronic conditions, such as diabetes. If you're a young primagravida—doctor-speak for first-timer—you won't be seen as often as an older primagravida, or a woman carrying twins. In a low-risk pregnancy, expect to see your carer once a month until Week 32, then every two weeks until the last month. In the last month, you'll be seen every week, and you'll probably be sick of the sight of doctors, nurses, and anything medical.

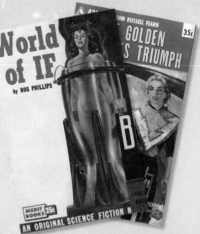

✳ In early pregnancy, Deirdre sometimes thought she might just as well be living in a test tube.

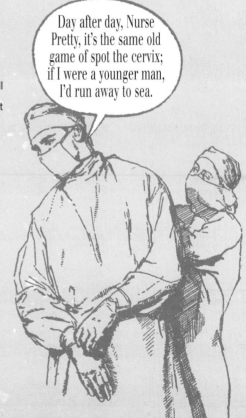

Day after day, Nurse Pretty, it's the same old game of spot the cervix; if I were a younger man, I'd run away to sea.

PEES ON CUE

Dignity is something you leave at the check-in desk of the delivery suite and collect around the time your child starts preschool, although you probably won't even notice you've misplaced it. That's because you'll be conditioned by months of being prodded and poked, peeing into plastic cups, and providing enough blood to start your own blood sausage factory. These are, indeed, testing times. Before long, you will pull up your sleeve at the sight of a white coat and be able to pee on demand.

It's just as well you have to pee all the time, because every nurse, midwife, physician, or obstetrician you see seems to hand you a little cup and ask for a sample. Urine provides a quick snapshot of your health, and warns of a number of potentially serious problems, so it is tested at every prenatal visit.

Message in a bottle

Urinary tract infections are very common. There is a one in ten chance that you'll get one at some stage, and if you do, there's a one in three chance of a repeat performance. Symptoms include a burning sensation when you pee, and wanting to go all the time. However, pregnancy does this to us anyway, so it can be easy to miss the signs. Cystitis and other urinary tract infections are easy to knock out with antibiotics, but if they are left untreated, bacteria can work their way back to the kidneys and cause pyelonephritis, the medical name for a kidney infection. This causes the same symptoms as a urinary tract infection, but with the added complications of fever and an ache in your side or the middle of your back. Pyelonephritis occurs in 1 or 2 percent of all pregnancies, and can trigger premature delivery. There's a suggestion that it might also increase the risk of abnormalities, although this hasn't really been proved.

Prevention is the best policy, and there is a lot you can do. Drink plenty of fluids, particularly cranberry juice, which contains plant chemicals that stop bacteria setting up home on the walls of your bladder and urinary tract.

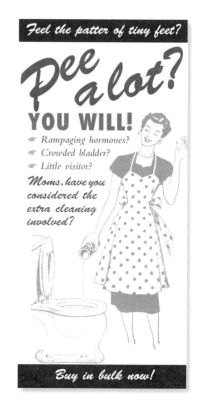

Feel the patter of tiny feet?

pee a lot?

YOU WILL!

☛ *Rampaging hormones?*
☛ *Crowded bladder?*
☛ *Little visitor?*

Moms, have you considered the extra cleaning involved?

Buy in bulk now!

Celia, a partner in a law firm, says, "The best bit of advice I got was not to put off going to the washroom and to squeeze out every last drop. It sounds simple enough, but there were times I'd be stuck in meetings, squirming around and crossing my legs and hey presto, a couple of days later I'd have cystitis. No meeting is that important!" Other tips are: wipe yourself from front to back, to avoid spreading fecal bacteria. Wear cotton underwear, avoid tight trousers, and go commando at bedtime. A lot of women find it also pays to restrict sugar intake: bacteria have a taste for sweet things, too.

Protein in the urine shows that your kidneys aren't coping very well, and this might need further investigation or monitoring. In the later stages of pregnancy, this can be a sign of pre-eclampsia or pregnancy-induced hypertension (PIH). We'll cover this later (*see pages 76–77*), but other symptoms include high blood pressure, swelling, and visual disturbances.

Sugar might show up in your urine as a result of normal changes caused by pregnancy hormones, or because of a more serious underlying problem such as diabetes. Millions of people in developed countries have Type 2 diabetes, which is associated with obesity and a diet of junk food, but the symptoms can be so mild they don't realize there is a problem. If you do have any blood sugar issues, the hormonal changes and extra workload of pregnancy will soon expose them. Latent diabetes can spring to life. You might develop a temporary glitch known as gestational diabetes, or a mild version of diabetes called glucose intolerance. As many as one in 20 women will get some degree of gestational diabetes. Symptoms include feeling very hungry and thirsty, a tendency to get thrush, and a rise in blood pressure. The treatment and potential risks depend on how badly your insulin response is affected.

❊ What do you mean I was supposed to do it in a plastic cup?

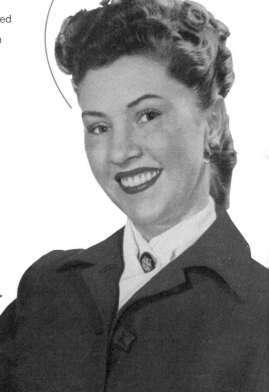

SWEET THING BALANCING BLOOD SUGAR

Insulin enables your body to burn blood sugar for fuel or convert it into stores of fat. Pregnancy increases the demand for fuel, so to ensure that there is always enough for the baby, the placenta pumps out body chemicals which slow down the way the mother's body uses insulin. This increases the amount of glucose that's sloshing around, and should ensure a perfect balance between the needs of mother and child. Like all balancing acts, it's a fine line between perfection and dejection.

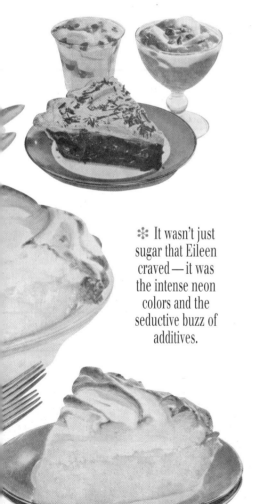

✳ It wasn't just sugar that Eileen craved—it was the intense neon colors and the seductive buzz of additives.

If you're not producing enough insulin, or it's not working hard enough, sugar will spill over into your urine, to show up on the little test strip your midwife or doctor dips into your pee. If sugar shows up on a single test, it's nothing to get stressed about; but if it appears on two urine tests in a row, your doctor will probably want you to have a glucose tolerance test. You'll have to starve for a few hours: the degree of deprivation will depend on your doctor. A small sample of blood will be taken to determine your fasting glucose level, which is the baseline that shows how much blood sugar there is usually. You'll then be given a measured dose of glucose, which usually means downing a bottle of Lucozade or some other energy drink. You'll have to hang around so that blood can be taken at timed intervals, typically one sample every hour for three hours. "By the time it's all over, you'll feel like a nauseated pincushion," warns Jodie, a 37-year-old mother of two, who has had blood sugar problems in both pregnancies.

Your fasting blood sugar level will fall by about 10 percent during the course of the pregnancy, and at various times hormones (including HPL, estrogen, and progesterone) can alter your insulin output, so the results of any glucose tolerance test will be interpreted in relation to your dates.

If a test confirms high blood sugar, don't panic, and don't punish yourself by trying to add up all the candy and cakes you've consumed. Poor diets might have contributed, but there are many other risk factors and indicators (*see box opposite*). The aim of any advice or treatment is to keep blood sugar levels within a fairly narrow band. Any action plan will depend on the degree of glucose intolerance you have. Often, exercise and simple dietary changes will make all the difference. Jodie says: "It wasn't quite as scary as it sounded. I was able to control my levels by cutting back on sugar and refined carbohydrates and eating more fiber, fruit, and vegetables. The toughest thing of all was giving up ice cream. Second time around, I was a lot more careful from the start, and although I had problems again, it wasn't so bad." If your glucose intolerance is severe, you may need medication or insulin injections. Diabetics who have previously been able to control their condition with diet alone usually find that they need insulin.

The bad news is that gestational diabetes appears to be on the increase, although no one can agree on how often it happens. Estimates range from one in 100 pregnancies to one in ten. The good news is that, in the vast majority of cases, blood sugar abnormalities resolve themselves once the baby is born. If you do get gestational diabetes, think of it as a wakeup call because it does mean that you are more likely to develop Type 2 diabetes when you get older.

If diabetes isn't controlled, particularly in the early stages of pregnancy, it can lead to neural tube defects and other abnormalities. When it develops later on in a pregnancy, it increases the likelihood of having a very big, or very small, baby, and of the baby having jaundice after delivery. Diabetes also increases the risk of complications such as urinary tract infections, thrush, pre-eclampsia, and excessive amniotic fluid. In extreme cases, the mother-to-be gets ketosis, which means she's burning reserves of muscle and fat instead of blood sugar, and releasing dangerous toxins in the process. The same thing happens on some high-protein, low-carbohydrate diets, which is why they're not as popular with doctors as they are with Hollywood stars.

RISK FACTORS

These include poor diet, a family history of diabetes; a history of miscarriage; a previous, unexplained stillbirth; having been a heavy baby; having a heavy baby in a previous pregnancy; being an older mother; and being seriously overweight.

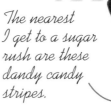

The nearest I get to a sugar rush are these dandy candy stripes.

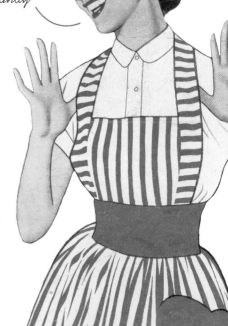

HYPERTENSION AND OTHER PRESSURES

"**D**ear diary: The house move is on hold, the boss is on my back about finding maternity coverage, and my feet are too swollen to fit into my expensive sandals..." Everyone says you should relax and enjoy your pregnancy, but there will be times when your body, baby, and buddies all seem to be conspiring to send your blood pressure into orbit. You know this is a no-no, but it's not easy to keep calm and contemplate your navel if it has turned itself inside out and you are in the grip of pregnancy hormones.

Blood pressure checks will happen every time you set foot inside a doctor's office, hospital, or health center. A lack of exercise, high sodium diets, and stressful lifestyles mean that a lot of women have problems with hypertension before pregnancy. This is called chronic hypertension ("chronic" meaning "long-term," not that it's really bad). A blood pressure check is the only way to diagnose this problem, because there are no noticeable symptoms. Chronic hypertension needs to be watched carefully, because it can— although it doesn't always—turn into toxemia or pre-eclampsia. Treatments might have to be adapted, too, as ACE inhibitors—a family of drugs often used to control hypertension—cannot be taken during pregnancy.

Really Madge, you must learn to avoid the stress of housework!

But Maris, it's your house I'm cleaning!

Highs and lows

Any form of hypertension, chronic or pregnancy-induced, involves added risks. It might restrict the flow of blood (and therefore oxygen and nutrients) to your baby and stall growth. It also increases the risk of the placenta coming away from the wall of the womb, which is known as placental abruption. This causes bleeding and may trigger a miscarriage.

When it comes to hypertension, there are a number of ways, both emotional and physical, that pregnancy can throw a wrench in the pumping works.

In the first few months, readings will dip as progesterone comes online and begins to stretch the veins and arteries. This ensures that your circulatory system expands to accommodate all the extra blood you are making to support your baby. It can also go straight to your head and cause dizziness and fainting.

Around the middle of the second trimester, your blood pressure should bottom out and then slowly rise again, until it gets back to where it was early in pregnancy. Sometimes it doesn't stop there. "My readings just kept on going," says Sissy, a 39-year-old bank employee. "We had a new manager and there was a lot of tension at work, so I was feeling completely strung out." Who doesn't at some time during pregnancy? But this pushes up adrenaline levels, and with them your blood pressure. Early baseline readings are important because they tell your doctor what's normal for you, and what's not. A blood pressure reading that is considered within an acceptable range for one woman might be cause for concern in another woman, so don't go swapping notes with other moms-to-be and put yourself into a panic. After all, this will only elevate your blood pressure.

A lot of women are surprised at how much blood pressure readings can fluctuate during pregnancy. Sissy says, "I noticed that my readings were often lower in the morning and then they were always a little higher when they were taken at the birth center." Physicians call this "white-coat hypertension," which is just another way of saying that hospitals can be scary places sometimes. Madeleine, who's 24 and having her first baby says, "I've always enjoyed yoga and I found that I could bring my blood pressure down by a few points with some of the meditation exercises. Before all my antenatal appointments, I would make a conscious decision to relax and take my head to another place. I'm sure it kept me out of the hospital on more than one occasion."

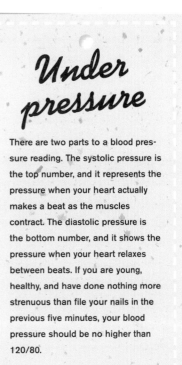

Under pressure

There are two parts to a blood pressure reading. The systolic pressure is the top number, and it represents the pressure when your heart actually makes a beat as the muscles contract. The diastolic pressure is the bottom number, and it shows the pressure when your heart relaxes between beats. If you are young, healthy, and have done nothing more strenuous than file your nails in the previous five minutes, your blood pressure should be no higher than 120/80.

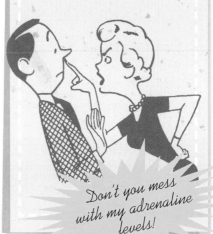

Don't you mess with my adrenaline levels!

When to worry

BUT DON'T PANIC!

Blood pressure is measured in millimeters of mercury—mmHg—and alarm bells will start ringing if your systolic pressure goes up by 30mmHg and the diastolic pressure rises by 15 mmHg, or the full reading tops 140/90. Figures like these add up to a warning of pre-eclampsia or toxemia. Other terms you might come across include gestational hypertension and pregnancy induced hypertension (PIH)—a catchall condition that includes gestational hypertension, pre-eclampsia, and toxemia. It turns up after the 20th week, though it is more common after the 30th, and should be monitored carefully. Sorry, that means more prenatal appointments. On the upside, PIH might not require treatment and usually goes away once the baby is born.

Pre-eclampsia

If your blood pressure is high and you have protein in your urine, you may be headed for the hospital and enforced bedrest. This combination is called pre-eclampsia or toxemia. Between 5 and 7 percent of women get pre-eclampsia, and it can lead to eclampsia. Eclampsia comes from the Greek word for lightning, and that's how it strikes: quickly, and with devastating results. Most cases are caught early, at the pre-eclamptic stage, but despite all these checks and the marvels of modern medicine, eclampsia is still the most common cause of death in childbirth. Other warning signs of pre-eclampsia are swelling, particularly in the hands and feet; blurred vision or seeing spots before your eyes; sudden weight gain; and splitting headaches.

Gestational hypertension won't necessarily move up a gear into pre-eclampsia, and pre-eclampsia doesn't automatically turn into eclampsia, but your doctor won't take any chances. If your blood pressure strays into the danger zone, you automatically become a high-risk patient. Treatment depends on how bad your readings are, the severity of the symptoms, and how far away your due date is.

SHBG

In the future, doctors might be able to predict who will develop toxemia by looking for a blood protein known as SHBG; women who get pre-eclampsia seem to be short of it.

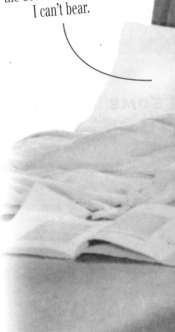

✳ I can live with the essential bed rest—it's the bed headboard that I can't bear.

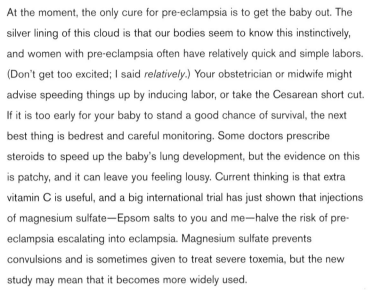

At the moment, the only cure for pre-eclampsia is to get the baby out. The silver lining of this cloud is that our bodies seem to know this instinctively, and women with pre-eclampsia often have relatively quick and simple labors. (Don't get too excited; I said *relatively*.) Your obstetrician or midwife might advise speeding things up by inducing labor, or take the Cesarean short cut. If it is too early for your baby to stand a good chance of survival, the next best thing is bedrest and careful monitoring. Some doctors prescribe steroids to speed up the baby's lung development, but the evidence on this is patchy, and it can leave you feeling lousy. Current thinking is that extra vitamin C is useful, and a big international trial has just shown that injections of magnesium sulfate—Epsom salts to you and me—halve the risk of pre-eclampsia escalating into eclampsia. Magnesium sulfate prevents convulsions and is sometimes given to treat severe toxemia, but the new study may mean that it becomes more widely used.

Very, very occasionally, pre-eclampsia, or eclampsia, can strike in labor or just after, so if your blood pressure has been high during pregnancy you should be checked more often in the postpartum period. This should include taking your blood pressure, testing urine for protein, and checking reflex responses. If you are not being monitored closely, ask why not.

What causes pre-eclampsia?

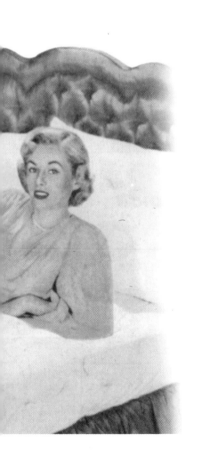

There are many different theories about what causes pre-eclampsia, including poor nutrition, genetics, and crossed wires in the mother's immune system. No one really knows for sure, and various conditions seem to increase the risk. These include: being a first-timer; being younger than 19 or older than 35; carrying twins, or more; having a close family member with PIH; diabetes; chronic kidney disease; and being overweight. Curiously enough, smokers are less likely to get pre-eclampsia, but when they do get it, they tend to get it worse.

BLOOD KNOWS

If the eyes are the windows to the soul, then the blood is the great big blabbermouth that spills the beans on what your body's been up to. There are no secrets with blood serum, and screening provides a quick snapshot of the state of your health, which is why your health provider is so eager to collect the stuff. Blood tests start at your first visit and might still be going on once your baby is born. They provide a great deal of information.

✳ Greta wondered
if a bloodcount was
as simple as
counting her
chickens...

One of the first tests your doctor or midwife will run is to find out what blood type you are and whether or not you have the "rhesus factor." If you are a negative blood group, and your baby's father is positive, it's not the perfect match in terms of blood types. If the mother is rhesus negative and the baby is rhesus positive, this sets off a chain reaction that can cause fetal anemia in subsequent pregnancies. The scene is set when rhesus positive blood from the fetus crosses the placenta and gets into the mother's bloodstream. This can happen during labor, a miscarriage, or a termination. When it does, the mother's immune system picks up the "alien" rhesus factor and goes on alert, producing antibodies to identify and attack the intruder. Like any allergic reaction, the symptoms don't start with the first exposure, but this sensitization means that the next time the mother's body finds blood cells with the rhesus factor, the immune system will attack anything—including a fetus—with the rhesus cells (*see box on opposite page*).

Safety shot

If you are rhesus negative, the key is to stop sensitization. Whenever there is a chance of fetal blood crossing the placenta, you will be given a shot of rhesus-immune globulin, also known as anti-D immunoglobulin. This destroys the fetal cells in your system and heads off the production of antibodies. It must be given within 72 hours, and the dose

ESSENTIALS

THE RHESUS FACTOR

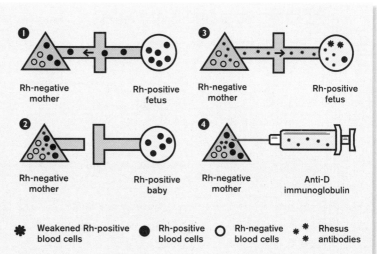

1 Rh-positive blood cells from fetus cross placenta to Rh-negative mother.

2 The mother produces antibodies after the Rh-positive blood has entered the bloodstream during delivery.

3 In a subsequent pregnancy the mother's rhesus antibodies will attack the Rh-positive blood of the growing baby, causing the blood disease.

4 Anti-D immunoglobulin is administered to prevent the production of rhesus antibodies.

Rh-negative mother	Rh-positive fetus
Rh-negative mother	Rh-positive fetus
Rh-negative mother	Rh-positive baby
Rh-negative mother	Anti-D immunoglobulin

* **Weakened Rh-positive blood cells**
● **Rh-positive blood cells**
○ **Rh-negative blood cells**
✱ **Rhesus antibodies**

will depend on how many fetal blood cells have gotten loose. It should protect you for around three months and it won't hurt your baby. Situations warranting a shot include any episodes of bleeding, and tests such as amniocentesis, which may release tiny amounts of fetal blood.

Moms-to-be who are rhesus negative have an extra blood test to see if they have already produced antibodies. Jacqui, a 28-year-old first-timer, says: "I knew that I was rhesus negative, so it was a worry. I was so relieved when the antibody test came back clear, showing I hadn't been sensitized. My physician gave me a shot of rhesus-immune globulin at 28 weeks, just in case, and then another shot just after my little girl was born, because she was rhesus positive." If blood tests show that you have already been sensitized, you will need regular checks of your antibody levels. If they start climbing, further tests, including amniocentesis, will be done to see what's happening to your baby. At delivery, doctors will be on standby to give the baby a blood transfusion to control jaundice. In extreme cases, a transfusion may be done while the baby is in the womb.

Hubbahubba! Our guys are really trashing those antibodies.

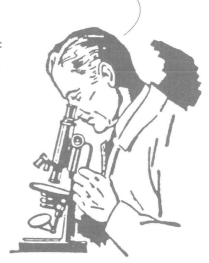

You can count on your blood

A full blood count—FBC on your notes—measures the number of red cells, white cells, and platelets (the glue that sticks everything together and makes blood clot). It also gives the lowdown on the proportion of your blood that is made up of red blood cells, and how much hemoglobin they contain.

A low number of red blood cells, or cells with a light load of hemoglobin, means that you're anemic. This is common after the first trimester, and can stall fetal development. Your blood is your baby's lifeline, delivering oxygen and nutrients and taking away carbon dioxide and other trash. To make sure there's enough blood for all this extra work, we make more. By the time your baby is ready to come out, you will have up to 50 percent more blood than you did at the beginning of your pregnancy. We need the mineral iron to make all this extra blood: it's an essential ingredient in hemoglobin, and if we're not getting enough, we become anemic. Babies need iron, too, and they grab theirs before you can, because in the last few months they have to stock the pantry with enough to last until they start eating solids. If an FBC shows that you are anemic, it should also say why, and what to do about it. If your red blood cells are small and pasty-looking, you need iron; if they are larger than normal and are just being lazy, then a vitamin deficiency is the most likely problem.

Extra white blood cells are a sign of infection or inflammation. There are a number of different kinds, and the type indicates whether the problem is bacterial or an allergic response. Having more extras than a Spielberg movie points to a bone marrow problem. If you don't have enough white blood cells, there is something wrong with your immune system or your diet is deficient to the point of malnutrition.

Doctors are also interested in blood chemistry. This is a check for all sorts of extras that don't necessarily add value, such as salts, enzymes, and proteins. If the wrong blood chemicals show up, it can be a sign of kidney, liver, bone, or muscle damage, or a temperamental thyroid.

✳ Fifty percent more blood! Can I trade it for a Tiffany pendant?

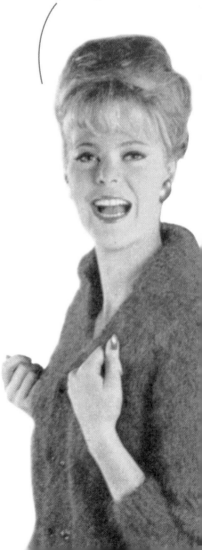

Down's syndrome

THE ODDS

Probability takes a turn for the worse around 35, and the odds shorten with every birthday— but don't make the mistake of thinking that Down's syndrome doesn't happen to younger moms, it does.

AGE	RISK
25	one in 1,500
30	one in 800
35	one in 350
36	one in 300
37	one in 200
38	one in 170
39	one in 140
40	one in 100
45	one in 30

Whether it's a lifestyle choice, career demands, or the sheer number of frogs you have to kiss to find Prince Charming, women are leaving it later to start a family. This advantage of this is that you're better prepared emotionally and financially, but it does increase the odds of complications such as Down's syndrome. Also known as trisomy 21 (because it's caused by having an extra copy of chromosome 21), Down's causes mental retardation, poor muscle tone, and easily recognizable facial characteristics. Over a third of Down's children also have heart abnormalities. Youth doesn't give any guarantees, but the risks of having a Down's baby increase as we get older (*see box at left*), probably because our eggs have been in the refrigerator a lot longer.

Risk charts can be scary, and you can get a better idea of your individual odds with a blood test for alpha fetoprotein (AFP). It's usually called an MSAFP (maternal serum alpha fetoprotein), although it may be combined with other checks and be called a "double" or "triple" test. A sample can be taken any time between 15 and 20 weeks, but Weeks 16 to 18 provide the best results. Low levels of AFP indicate an increased risk of a chromosomal problem such as Down's, while elevated levels are a clue to spina bifida and other neural tube defects. It's important to remember that these are clues, not a definite diagnosis. "My MSAFP came up low risk," says Fiona, a 36-year-old mom of two. "A friend who was pregnant was told her risk was really high, but she went ahead anyway. My daughter was born with Down's and my friend's baby was fine. The odds of it happening were probably a million to one, but it happened, and when it happens to you, it can be very, very hard to handle." There are also other defects that MSAFP won't reveal. The other downside of MSAFP testing is that you might have to wait a week or so for the results, and by the time you have the test, the pregnancy is quite advanced. Other tests, such as CVS, amniocentesis, and the nuchal fold, can be done earlier: more on those later (*see pages 83–87*).

SCAN DO FIRST FAMILY PHOTOS

Ultrasound scans mean we can have snapshots of our babies for the family album long before they are born. Seeing your baby for the first time will be an incredible experience for mom and dad, but don't expect friends and family to find these fuzzy images as fascinating as you do. Ultrasound techniques and technology are improving all the time, and an embryo is visible as early as six weeks from conception. The amniotic sac can be seen even earlier, particularly if the scan is done vaginally.

Timetables vary, but scans are routinely done quite early on to confirm dates; at around 18 weeks to look for abnormalities, such as NTDs, and to make sure that all the internal organs are in the right place; and in the final weeks to check that your baby isn't a bighead and likely to get stuck on the way out. Extra scans might be also be carried out to monitor a high-risk pregnancy; to check that the cervix is staying firmly shut; to track down an IUD that didn't do its job; to find the fetus for amniocentesis or CVS; to count how many guests are on board; to see where the placenta has stuck itself; and to see how much fluid there is for your baby to splash around in.

Seeing is believing

Take along the tissues, and your partner or a good friend, for your first scan, because it can be an emotional experience. The picture quality varies depending on the equipment, the operator, how much pee you have in your bladder at the time, and where the baby is. On a good day, you might see him or her sucking a thumb or fiddling with the umbilical cord. If the scan is being done externally (and most are), the operator will want you to have a full bladder. When appointments aren't running to schedule, which is often the case, this is the only discomfort you should feel.

For the scan, you'll lie on your back and have your belly basted with more goop than a Thanksgiving turkey. This gel acts as a conductor. A small unit is then moved across your tummy, sending out soundwaves that bounce

ESSENTIALS

THE ULTRASOUND

Ultrasound (also known as sonography) scans can be done at any time to check the development of the fetus or for multiple pregnancies.

around your womb. As the echoes come back, they are turned into images on a screen the size of a TV. When the scan is done internally, a small probe is inserted into the vagina. It's too small to be described as a dildo (tough), but you might have to brace yourself against a fit of the giggles as the operator slips a condom onto it. "I had a cervical cerclage [see page 53], so I lost count of how many internal scans I had, but it used to crack me up every time," says Dawn, a 36-year-old marketing executive. "I'm not sure who was more embarrassed, me or the guy doing the scan."

The clarity of ultrasound images is improving all the time, and the images are being used for a greater number of purposes. Sharp-eyed scanners have noticed that babies with Down's syndrome get it in the neck—literally. When the fetus is only a few weeks old, it has a fold of skin at the nape of the neck that is filled with fluid. It is called the nuchal fold, and it can hold clues to chromosome faults. The more fluid there is in the nuchal fold, the greater the risk of Down's syndrome. Like AFP, it doesn't give a definite yes or no, but it gives odds accurate enough to make a racetrack bookie turn green with envy. The advantage of the nuchal fold scan is that it's quick, you get a ballpark figure right away, and it's noninvasive. It's not as accurate as amniocentesis or CVS, but it can be done as early as 11 weeks, so if the odds aren't in your favor you can always have the other tests later on.

Ultrasound, or sonography as it's sometimes called, has been used for more than 30 years, and seems to be safe. However, there is no guarantee that side effects won't show up in the future, so ultrasound should be used only when absolutely necessary, and never just to get a few more baby photos.

✳ Look, Eugene, the little zygote's got my nose!

✳ He sure has, Walt. And your glasses.

AMNIOCENTESIS, PUBS, AND CVS

There are times when you will need more information than blood tests and ultrasound scans can provide, and your doctor might suggest more accurate, but more intrusive, tests such as amniocentesis, chorionic villus sampling, or percutaneous umbilical cord sampling (also known as cordocentesis). That's all a bit of a mouthful in one go, so now that everyone's been formally introduced, we'll call them amnio, CVS, and PUBS.

✣ Wearing his 'n' her sweaters doesn't mean you need to be tested for twins.

All three tests involve sticking a needle into the womb and taking out a tiny sample for analysis. Amnio scoops up fetal cells in amniotic fluid, CVS takes fetal cells from a tiny bit of the chorion (a thin membrane that becomes part of the placenta), and PUBS takes blood from the umbilical cord. Because these tests involve fetal cells, they give a much clearer picture of what's going on in your womb. They can be used to screen for a number of inherited conditions, including: sickle-cell anemia; most types of cystic fibrosis; Tay-Sachs; thalassemia; Duchenne's muscular dystrophy (see box on page 87); and chromosomal problems such as Down's syndrome. Amnio and CVS will tell you the gender of the fetus. This is more important than a matter of color schemes if you carry an X-linked genetic disorder such as hemophilia, which emerges only in males. PUBS can be used to take blood from the mother's side of the placenta, so it can also be used to keep an eye on how much oxygen is getting through and to monitor very bad cases of rhesus incompatibility. It is now more widely used than fetoscopy, which uses a tiny probe mounted with lights and a camera to spy on the baby and collect tissue samples.

The whole point of an amniotic sac is that it's shut tight, keeping the fetus cocooned and protected from the world outside, with all its bacteria and bugs. Anything that involves breaking this seal or having a rummage around inside the womb carries an element of risk. The chances of something going wrong are very low—less than 1 percent in the case of amnio—but they have to be considered. A great deal depends on the skill of the person doing the amnio, so it's well worth asking their individual batting average. We loved it when one less than bashful obstetrician talked through the relative risks, and then boasted, "But that's the national average, and I'm not average! I'm *much* better than that!" At any other time, we'd have been itching to bring him down a peg or two, but at that moment we put him on a pedestal instead. This is just what you want to hear from the person who's about to stick a needle into your belly.

IN THE KNOW

If tests reveal a problem, genetic counseling will give you a much clearer understanding of the risks and implications. Don't avoid tests because your religious beliefs mean that a termination is out of the question. Some conditions can be corrected in the womb, or shortly after birth.

What happens next

Most amnio is done purely on the basis of age. No one can agree on exactly what age that is, but if you are 35 years old or older, you will probably be offered one. For the test itself, you'll probably have to strip and slip into one of those ghastly gowns that never quite meet at the back. If you're lucky, you may need only to pull up your top half and lower the bottom half. Although ultrasound is used as a guide during amnio, you will be asked to have a pee before the test, which might seem a bit of a contradiction. A full bladder makes for better ultrasound pictures, but an empty bladder is better for amnio. Your stomach will get a quick once over with an antiseptic wipe, and you may be given a local anesthetic. Don't be surprised, or go into a panic, if you're not given one. Many doctors don't bother, arguing that the injection itself is as painful, if not more so, than the momentary prick of the needle going through the skin. This might sound strange, and slightly sadistic, but it's true. Women who

❋ Just because I'm a woman of a certain age in a ghastly gown doesn't mean I need amnio...I'm not actually pregnant!

✳ With all this amniotic fluid about, a girl can't afford to take any chances!

are so chicken that Colonel Sanders should have coated them in his secret recipe years ago, can vouch for the fact that you don't need an anesthetic. Once the needle is through the top layer, which is where all the nerve endings are located, you don't actually feel a thing. I speak from experience on this one. I was completely horrified when my obstetrician told me that I wouldn't need an anesthetic, but the toughest bit of the test by far was watching the ultrasound monitor and seeing a needle the size of a baseball bat heading toward a beautiful little baby—my beautiful little baby.

Two or three spoonfuls of amniotic fluid—a tiny fraction of the amount your baby is floating in—are sucked out through the syringe and sent off to a lab, where they are planted in a culture dish to grow. These cells are then used to identify any fetal abnormalities. Some problems show up in a matter of days, but it may be three nail-biting weeks before you have the full picture. Amnio is usually done between Weeks 15 and 18. If an abnormality is detected, you might want to terminate the pregnancy, or you might feel that you can cope and that your child will still have a reasonable quality of life. This is a decision that only you and your partner can make, and you shouldn't feel pressured either way. If you do, complain—very loudly.

CVS and PUBS

CVS works along similar lines to amnio, but is done earlier in the pregnancy, at around nine weeks—when a termination would be much less traumatic—and the needle might be inserted through the vagina to remove fetal tissue. The chorion villis, which is being sampled, is the beginnings of the placenta. Like the amniotic fluid, it contains fetal cells that can be grown and examined for abnormalities. In terms of the

ESSENTIALS

GENE GENIES—INHERITED CONDITIONS

Hereditary illnesses are handed down in one of three ways: recessive inheritance, dominant inheritance, and X-linked. With recessive inheritance, either the guy or the gal has a dud gene, but it can be passed on. If your partner carries a faulty version of the same gene, there is a one in four chance that you will both pass on the dud.

SICKLE CELL ANEMIA

A form of anemia in which the red blood cells are weaker and sickle-shaped. This causes blockages that deprive organs and tissues of oxygen.

TAY-SACHS

A disease, usually carried by Ashkenazi Jews, characterized by mental and physical retardation.

CYSTIC FIBROSIS

A disease of the exocrine glands, which affects the pancreas, respiratory system, and sweat glands.

DUCHENNE'S MUSCULAR DYSTROPHY

A disorder characterized by general weakness and wasting of skeletal muscle.

THALASSEMIA

A blood disorder that results in a decrease in the amount of hemoglobin formed.

procedure, the only difference between amnio and PUBS is the target: In PUBS it's the cord, not the amniotic fluid. A tiny sample of the baby's blood is taken for analysis. The advantage of PUBS is that it gives quick, accurate results, but as far as your fetus is concerned it's a much more intrusive procedure.

For any of these tests, take someone along to hold your hand and help you get home. You should lie down for the rest of day, and possibly the next few days as well. The puncture mark on your belly might feel tender, and some women get mild cramps afterward.

Occasionally, something goes seriously wrong, but this is extremely rare. With amnio, there is a 0.5–1 percent risk of miscarriage, fetal death, bleeding, infection, or a leak of amniotic fluid. With CVS, there is a slightly higher risk of miscarriage. If the placental tissue has been taken from the mother's side, a false result is possible. One study suggests that CVS can damage developing limbs. The jury is still out on this one, but you should be aware of the risks. PUBS carries significant risks and is done only when absolutely necessary.

FETAL CHECKS

By the time you've made it to your first prenatal appointment, your baby's heart is already beating and, depending on the equipment used, might be audible. Eavesdropping is called auscultation, and it will happen during every visit. Other fetal checks include putting the squeeze on your pregnant belly (it helps if the person doing it has warm hands—don't be afraid to ask) and, later on in pregnancy, monitoring the daily number of kicks that Junior aims at your belly.

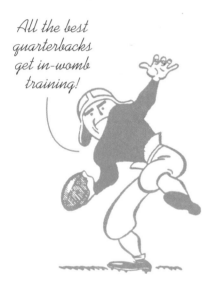

All the best quarterbacks get in-womb training!

PALPATION

This is the name for the prodding and squeezing of your pregnant belly, which enables your doctor to check the size and position of your uterus and baby; how many babies are in there; how much fluid is sloshing around; and whether the head is "engaged."

The most basic baby bugging kit is a little trumpet-shaped instrument known as Pinard's fetal stethoscope. The big end is put on your tummy, and your carer sticks the little end in his or her ear. The next model up is a little electrical unit that is held against your tummy, picking up and amplifying the heartbeat. The state-of-the-art supersnoop is a hospital monitor with electrodes attached to a couple of bands, which are strapped around your belly. This monitors and records both the heart rate and the contractions or fetal movements. The baby's heart beats very rapidly in the womb, between 110 and 160 beats per minute, so it will sound a bit like a galloping horse.

If you suspect that something is wrong, or you start to bleed, you will probably be trussed up and monitored to let the doctors look for any signs of fetal distress. Some hospitals also like to do a routine 20-minute session just to make sure that everything is OK, while others prefer to monitor women throughout labor. There are different schools of thought on this. Some studies have shown that if you are continually monitored in labor, there's a greater chance of intervention. Some physicians and midwives also argue that continual monitoring puts the machine in charge, instead of a person who has been there, and done it, plenty of times before. It's worth asking about the policy that your doctor or birth center has on monitoring in labor, and thinking through the implications. You might want to put down some ground rules of your own in your birthplan.

BUT DON'T PANIC!

Get a kick out of life

When it's your first pregnancy, you should start to feel the baby move between Weeks 18 and 20. At first, it's a funny, fluttery feeling, a bit like having real butterflies in your stomach, and you may not realize what it is. Women who've had a baby before know what's coming, and are able to feel these faint movements (called "quickening") as early as 16 weeks. As your baby grows and starts dreaming of becoming a fullback, you can't miss the movements. If you happen to be in a position that your baby doesn't like, be prepared for a sharp elbow in the kidneys. Later in the pregnancy, the acrobatics get so intense that these movements can be clearly seen, and it may look as if you've got a litter of playful kittens down your jumper.

One way to make sure everything's on track is to record these movements on a kick chart. You should feel something going on at least ten times a day. The trick is to find out what schedule your baby is on, and be alert to any changes of routine. Every baby has his or her favorite time for a workout, but babies tend to keep teenage hours and often save frenetic activity for the evenings. As a general rule, you should start logging activity on your kick chart at nine in the morning, and keep a record for the next 12 hours. However, if you have a real night owl who rarely wants to play before sundown, start your chart later in the day to make sure that it covers the period of peak activity.

Alarm bells should start ringing if it takes your baby longer each day to clock up ten kicks. Movements become more restricted as the baby grows and starts running out of space, but you should always feel something. If there's no hint of activity within any ten-hour period, or the pattern changes dramatically, call your doctor or hospital right away, no matter what time of the day or night it is. If you're very close to your due date, this could be a clue to get your bags ready: many women find their baby goes quiet and has a bit of a rest just before labor begins.

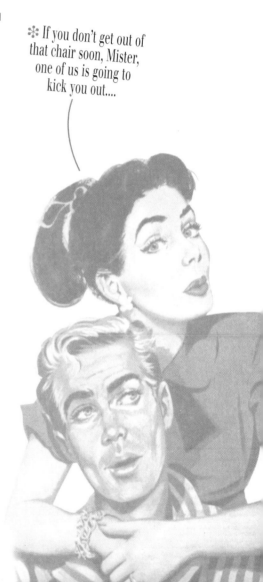

❋ If you don't get out of that chair soon, Mister, one of us is going to kick you out....

Just let me know if you want a hand with anything.

Sex,
exercise, and food

These three lynchpins of life before you got pregnant remain just as important now that you're headed for motherhood. "Sensible" is the best word to use in the context of exercise and food to keep you well *and* happy. If you've never been perfect (leave that to your mother's best friend's daughter), there's no reason to start now. Sex is another matter—nothing is as various as the pregnant woman's response to the idea of sex, and you'll find the sheer diversity of experiences entertaining.

✳ *At last! All the sex you want—and some of the chocolate—but none of the guilt.*

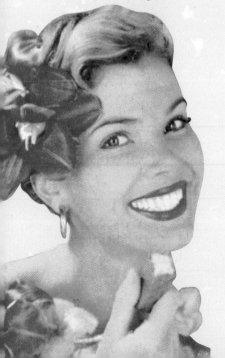

When you consider that it was sex that got us into all this in the first place, it's amazing that some pregnancy books feel the need to explain how it's done. Hey, I think we worked that one out! Sex during pregnancy can be incredibly erotic, erratic, or even both at once. For some women, once a week is more than enough; for others, once a day doesn't even come close. Some women can go into orgasm overdrive, and keep coming back for more.

Terms like "normal" are fine when you're talking about shampoo and tampons, but when it comes to sex in pregnancy, they're as helpful as a heavy blow with a blunt instrument. "Normal" reactions to sex during pregnancy vary from feeling positively puritan to playacting the porn star. If you don't believe us, check out a few Internet chatrooms about pregnancy: you might find answers to questions that you'd never dreamed of asking. "Do you think my husband would mind if we didn't have any sex for the next year or so?"—Honey, do you really need an answer? "The doctor said we shouldn't have vaginal sex, so is anal OK?"—It depends on why you've been advised to keep your legs crossed, but there are good reasons for putting an "Exit Only" sign over the back door, including the risk of crossinfection, and the possibility of injury because of changing muscle tone.

YES!! YES!! NO!!

Trimester timewarps

Timing can make a lot of difference, too. In the first trimester, a great deal of women find that their sex drive slips into neutral, or even reverse. This is hardly surprising when you consider the amount of time you spend puking, sleeping, and pinching yourself just to make sure that you really are pregnant. "I've usually got a good appetite when it comes to sex. On that score, I'd definitely say that I am more of a three-course meal girl than a snacker," says Sally, a 29-year-old nurse-midwife. "But sex was the last thing on my mind in those early weeks. Maybe it was because I could sense that my boyfriend was getting cold feet about the pregnancy, or perhaps it was the constant tiredness. Whatever it was, I just didn't want to know."

The risk of miscarriage is at its highest in these early weeks, and there are a lot of test results to wait for, and worry over. All of these factors, plus the pregnancy hormones percolating through your body, may mean that you feel more protective than a Jewish momma in a Woody Allen movie. Letitia and her husband had already had four attempts at IVF when she got pregnant and she wasn't taking any chances. "My physician said there was no reason why we shouldn't have sex, but we just weren't comfortable with the idea. The memory of all those appointments, and weeks of waiting for what had turned out to be bad news, was the ultimate passion killer. I didn't want to take any risks at all, and Ricky felt the same way. I don't think he could have gotten an erection if he'd tried, not even with Viagra. Going without sex wasn't an issue because we both wanted to abstain—and after Jolie was born, we had great fun catching up."

It's during the middle trimester, from Week 14 to Week 26, that you're most likely to get turned on more often than a light switch. Don't be surprised if you suddenly develop the appetite (if not the body and wardrobe) of Samantha from *Sex and the City*. It doesn't happen to

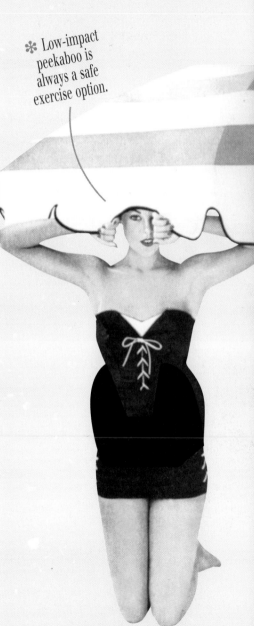

❋ Low-impact peekaboo is always a safe exercise option.

everyone, but it's a lot more common than some pregnancy books, and doctors, tend to suggest. "It's not the sort of thing anyone mentions," says Madeleine, 24. "And it's certainly not the sort of thing you can ask your mom about, but when I did accidentally let something slip at my antenatal class there was pandemonium. Half the women thought I was completely crazy and were shaking their heads in disbelief, while the other half were screeching, 'You too?' Afterward, one of the other ladies came up to me and said, 'Wow, I'm so glad you said that. I thought there was something wrong with me.' "

Going down?

When you look back at old medical journals and pregnancy books, it's curious to see what the so-called experts have suggested about sex over the years. Given the emphasis on fears and fellatio that used to color most advice and much research—even as recently as the supposedly swinging sixties—it's no wonder that so many women used to say they didn't like sex during pregnancy. For starters, there were dire warnings that cunnilingus could kill you. There is actually a tiny grain of truth to this one: in theory, a particularly energetic session, combined with the general softening up of your vagina and circulatory system as a result of pregnancy hormones, could cause an embolism—a tiny air bubble in the bloodstream—which could go straight to your head and block up a bit of brain. It's possible, but it's about as likely as winning the lottery or landing a place on the next moon-shot.

The only real difference in terms of oral sex during pregnancy is that things look and taste a bit different down there. Dildos are OK, but you might feel happier with a slimline version than a Mr. Whopper. And don't forget to give it a good wash afterward. Given that so many pregnancy books used to be written by men perhaps it's not so

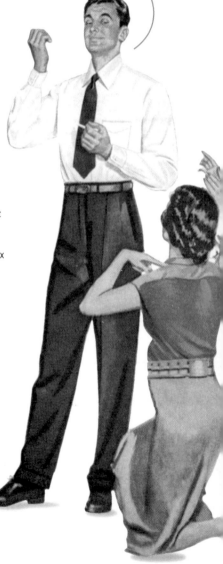

✳ You first, flower girl; see you upstairs as soon as I've finished my between-the-acts cigarette.

surprising that a lot of advice about oral sex used to end on a reassuring note, explaining to women that while cunnilingus was risky it was perfectly safe to give your man head. Thanks guys, that's really big of you.

By the third trimester, if you've got the stamina for it, sex is reduced to a series of logistical puzzles. Your partner might begin to feel like a dolphin trying to do it with a blue whale. For most women, the biggest attraction is the hope that sex could start labor. Once you're on the home stretch, good sex can trigger contractions. (Unsatisfactory sex won't do much at all—so no change there, then.) Any orgasm makes your womb contract and wind up like a clockwork toy, getting ready for the big release. During pregnancy, orgasm can be delayed, and the womb often takes longer to relax completely. This prolongs the fun, but it can be a bit spooky the first time it happens. Semen is packed with prostaglandins, and female orgasm releases a hit of oxytocin: these are two of the hormones that get labor moving. However, in general, any postcoital contractions are just a little turbulence on the magic carpet ride. Labor only follows lust when it was on the schedule anyway.

Size does matter   BIG FUN

But hey, it's impressive that you're even thinking about it! By this stage, you'll have the grace and flexibility of a supertanker. Demi Moore may have posed as an erotic vamp for the cover of *Vanity Fair* when she was pregnant, but it's our bet that she wasn't coming across for Bruce by then. It's extremely hard to get the hots when your body begins to feel like a size eight frock stretched over a size 18 frump. Then there are all those extra-seductive attributes, like hemorrhoids, indigestion, swollen ankles, and nosebleeds. These are great for softening up the psyche and convincing you that labor can't really be that bad, but when it comes to foreplay, they have all the erotic appeal of a double epidural.

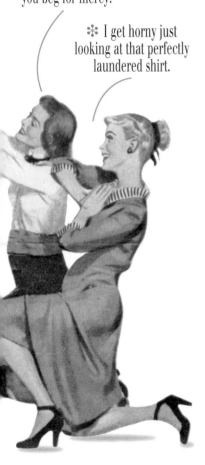

✳ Me next, big boy —
I'll polish your nails 'til
you beg for mercy!

✳ I get horny just
looking at that perfectly
laundered shirt.

Assuming that you're up for it, and he is, too, then your biggest problem is positioning. This requires more thought than a UN seating plan. By the beginning of the third trimester, lying flat on your back may make you feel dizzy because the large uterus can compress the inferior vena cava and decrease blood flow to the placenta. Wedging a pillow under one hip is enough to relieve this. All this weight has much the same effect as someone standing on the hose while you're trying to water the garden: the flow stops, or splutters to a sprinkle.

Positions that avoid pressure on your belly and boobies are usually the most comfortable. "Until I was pregnant, I'd never been a big fan of doing it doggy style," says Jessica, who's 41 and having her first baby. "Toward the end, it was the only position we could manage. The only thing I did notice was that if we had sex too soon after I'd eaten, it gave me dreadful heartburn. I know they talk about having the hots for someone when you're in the mood for sex, but that's heat you can do without." Another position that is likely to hit the spot is lying side by side like a couple of spoons in a drawer. There's no bulge to negotiate and no problems with blood flow. Girl on top works well, too, as you can control the action and the degree of penetration. Don't be afraid to sit down on the job: if you do it right on the edge of the bed, your partner can kneel in front of you (the perfect position for any man, don't you think?).

Finding a position that provides maximum pleasure with minimum pressure is a matter of experimentation, so don't be afraid to try out something new. You won't be up for major sexual gymnastics, but you might strike it lucky with a few orchestral maneuvers in the dark. At this stage of the game, the best sex aid to have is a pillow, or lots of pillows. Use them to prop up bulges, and support bits of the body that are getting tired and heavy.

Oh Winthrop, honey, come back — my headache's gone now!

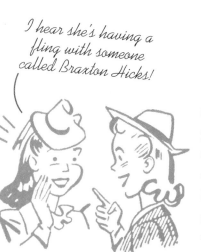

I hear she's having a fling with someone called Braxton Hicks!

What a workout!

Apart from the fact that it's a whole lot of fun, there are other reasons to have plenty of sex during pregnancy. Having an orgasm exercises the same uterine muscles that you'll use to push your baby out, so anything that strengthens and tones them is a bonus. Later on, this may start mini contractions, but it won't start labor. Orgasms will also make you more aware of your pelvic floor muscles and ensure that you're clinching the right bits when you're doing your Kegels (*see pages 98–101*).

WHEN TO SAY NO

Warning signals

Basically, sex is safe so long as neither of you is playing away from home, you're not leaking amniotic fluid or have broken your waters, and there are no other risk factors. However, there are times when doctors advise crossing your legs and taking cold showers. If you've miscarried before, it's best to skip sex in the early months, particularly around the times your period would be due. Most physicians also suggest saying no, just for a day or two, after invasive tests such as amnio or CVS. You'll probably be advised to avoid any action if you've got an incompetent cervix or need a cervical cerclage. Any sign of bleeding requires an immediate exit and prompt medical advice. Orgasmic contractions and Braxton Hicks practice contractions are usually unproblematic, but if you've gone into premature labor at any time and have been pulled back from the brink, you'll be advised to abstain.

No thanks, we're expecting

Most couples don't have to worry about these physical problems, but it's the mental ones that can really ground your libido. Just as women vary in their attitudes toward sex during pregnancy, so do guys. Some can't quite believe their luck at their partner's newfound lust for, er, lust, and enjoy every moment of it, which might explain why some dads-to-be walk around with permanent grins. Others are shagged into submission and may be surprised, and even a little embarrassed, to discover that you really can have too much of a good thing, even when that good thing is sex. "I'm like a rabbit in heat when I'm pregnant," says Miriam, a mother of three. "I wake up horny and stay that way all day, even when we've had sex and it's been great. I sometimes think it's nature's way of compensating guys for the weeks, maybe months, after the baby's born, when you don't have the inclination, the energy, or the opportunity to have sex."

Some men adore all this libidinous attention, but others get incredibly twitchy at the mere thought of sticking anything "up there." It's OK guys, it won't wake the baby! Jessica, a down-to-earth 41-year-old, admits she found this really hard to handle: "In the first few weeks, I wasn't fussed about not having sex. I had morning sickness most of the day, not really badly, but enough to put you off the idea of sex. Once I got into the second trimester, things really changed. I felt really good, super-charged, and screaming for sex. At first, Peter kept avoiding the subject, or making excuses, but after a while we couldn't ignore it any more. We'd always had a really good sex life and Peter's lack of interest really upset me. I thought it was because he didn't fancy me any more, and I even suspected him of having an affair. That wasn't the problem at all; he was just terrified of hurting me or the baby."

Then there's the whole "mother" thing. Now that you're on the way to becoming one, your other half might be looking for a pedestal to put you on. For some men, "moms" are all about apple pie and wholesome values, and they couldn't possibly indulge in anything as messy as sex. Well, they did once, but it was such a long time ago that their sons think it doesn't count.

Oedipus aside, mothers are for nurturing rather than nookie in most cultures, and there might be some big psychological hurdles to jump before you both feel like jumping into bed. Don't get us wrong: there's nothing wrong with calling it quits at a cuddle, so long as that's what you both want. However, if one of you is gagging for sex while the other gags at the mere thought, things are guaranteed to get more tense than a Florida recount. It can be incredibly hard—literally— when you're out of sync sexually, and it's important to try to reach some sort of compromise.

If your man's worried about penetration, it's a good idea to suggest he talks to your

✳ Darling, it's very sweet of you, but that's not really the kind of package I wanted to unwrap.

ESSENTIALS

STDS IN PREGNANCY

Sexually transmitted diseases in pregnancy take on even more difficult consequences. Symptoms include an unpleasant smelling discharge, abdominal pain, pain when you pee, and blisters or spots. HIV, hepatitis, and secondary stage syphilis (now extremely rare) can cross the placental barrier. If you're HIV-positive, drug treatments are available to cut the risk of transmission to your baby, and you'll probably be advised to have a C-section. Babies can be protected from Hepatitis B with an injection after delivery, and syphilis can be treated with antibiotics during pregnancy. STDs can increase the risk of an early arrival, but the biggest risk comes during delivery. Gonorrhoea and chlamydia, for example, can cause eye infections, and active genital herpes can spread to the baby once it leaves the safety of the womb. Then there are the relationship angles. If one of you is playing away, this suggests that your relationship isn't entirely rosy. Talk things through now, and make a commitment to stick together on terms you're both happy with.

physician to get the facts, not the fears. Alternatively sit him down with a pile of pregnancy books (including this one at the top of the pile!) and mark the chapters that talk about the safety of sex—and preferably not the ones that suggest blow-jobs for the boys and very little else. Pregnancy websites are another good way to air this sort of problem. They're reassuringly anonymous and apart from the odd whacko, most Internet chatrooms and bulletin boards are populated by real people with real solutions to real problems.

For a do-it-yourself approach, try suggesting a little mutual mouth-to-organ resuscitation, or put on a floorshow with a dildo. If you're lucky, your man will pluck up the courage to join in, and if you're not, you'll still have a good time. Try talking to girlfriends who've been there, and who kept on doing it through pregnancy. A similar locker-room chat might be all that's needed to stiffen your partner's resolve. Whatever you do, keep talking. Cracks in a relationship during pregnancy have a nasty habit of turning into gaping great chasms once parents are faced with the added pressure of a demanding new baby. And you never know, if you try talking dirty, it might just do the trick.

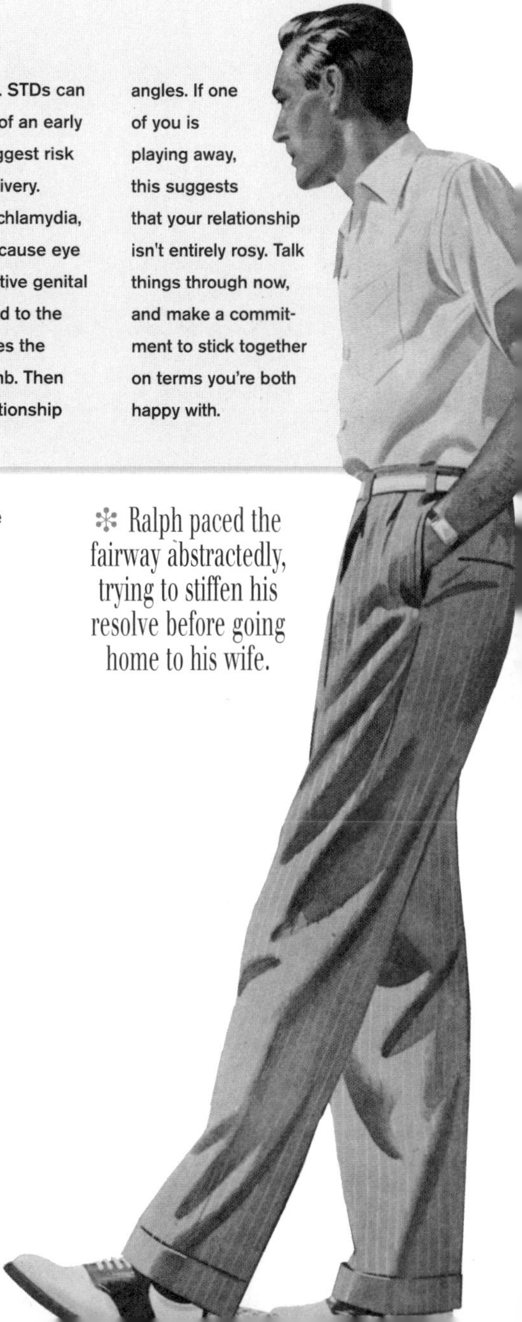

❊ Ralph paced the fairway abstractedly, trying to stiffen his resolve before going home to his wife.

THE PELVIC FLOOR   HOW TO KEEP IT IN GOOD SHAPE

When it comes to sex during pregnancy, kama sutra acrobatics might be out of the question, but there is a workout from the same school that every pregnant woman should practice: pelvic floor exercises. A well-toned pelvic floor will do wonders for your sex life and help prevent tearing during delivery. Pelvic floor exercises are also known as Kegel exercises, after the doctor who supposedly invented them, but they've actually been around for centuries.

In some Asian cultures, all girls are encouraged to do these exercises to improve their performance in the bedroom. As a result, their pelvic floor muscles recover faster after the baby has been born. In the West, we've still got a lot to learn, and some women need a map to find the right muscles. Make sure you get the map to give you some idea of where the muscles are, and put in more roadwork than Sylvester Stallone in a *Rocky* movie, because if you don't you'll turn into a dribbling wreck—literally!

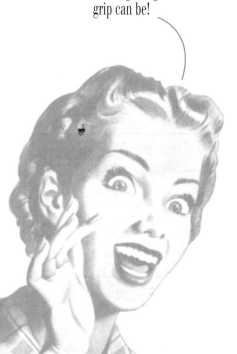

❊ Hey, girls! I've just discovered how much fun getting a grip can be!

Don't be a slouch

The pelvic floor consists of a series of muscles that hold all your organs and sexy bits in place, and control the outlet valves when you have a pee or a poop. The biggest of these muscles is slung, just like a hammock, from each side of the pelvis. Then there are smaller supporting players that run around the vagina and anus and hook everything up to your coccyx—the tail stump at the base of your spine, which is sometimes called a monkey stump—and other bony bits.

The pelvic floor muscles tighten and contract to give you a good time when you have an orgasm, and they also protect and support your womb, bladder, and rectum. Like all muscles, they are softened up by pregnancy hormones. If your pelvic floor is weak, which is most likely if you've had a baby before, you might feel as if the baby is about to fall out, particularly if you have to run or hurry. During pregnancy and labor, these muscles are

SEX TOY

You can buy toys, like little metallic balls or egg shapes, to put inside your vagina to keep your mind on the job while doing your pelvic floor exercises. There's no evidence that they make the workout more effective, but if they remind you to do your exercises and make them more pleasurable, there's no harm in trying them out.

✳ Sadie stayed as cool as a cucumber even after a marathon session polishing her pelvic floor.

stretched further than a bungee cord, and if you haven't done your exercises they will probably have all the bounce of a balloon filled with water. Subsequently, your sex life might suffer because you'll have lost a lot of your grip, and you might start to spring a leak whenever you cough, sneeze, laugh, or can't find a john the minute you want one. Trust us, this is one bit of homework you need to do thoroughly.

How to find your pelvic floor

The simplest way to find your pelvic floor muscles is to try to stop the flow when you're having a pee. Another way is to sit on a chair, put your fingers under your bottom, and place your thumb in your love canal (vagina!), pointing backward. Try to squeeze your thumb without moving your butt cheeks or tummy. Once you've found the front bit of the pelvic floor muscle, try to locate the bit at the back by stopping a bowel motion. You should be able to tighten these two areas independently, although this sometimes takes a little practice and at first you might find that they work together.

This all makes it sound a great deal more complicated than it really is, but if you aren't completely sure that you've got it right, have a bit of fun by trying a bit of practice on your partner. You don't even have to tell him what you're up to; the smile on his face will probably give the game away. "A lot of the pregnancy books make pelvic floor exercises sound so clinical and boring," says Maria, a 32-year-old mom of two. "It's a lot more fun to try gripping your guy, if you know what I mean. You'll probably get some appreciative feedback, too." If you're really baffled, ask your midwife or the hospital physical therapist for some help. OK, I know that some people find this sort of stuff embarrassing, but believe me, you're so used to being poked and prodded down there by this stage in your pregnancy that there will be barely any room for embarrassment left.

If you don't pay attention to keeping your pelvic floor muscles in good shape, you could also store up a whole host of problems for subsequent pregnancies and later life. When your ovaries shut down and you go into menopause, plummeting hormone levels will make all of these muscles even looser. This is why so many old ladies—and a few ladies who aren't as old as you might think—have to wear incontinence pads. It's not a fashion statement that we would recommend. Even if you have a take-it-or-leave-it attitude to exercise, and usually end up leaving it, you should definitely make an exception in this case.

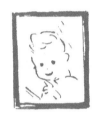
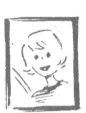
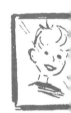

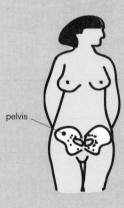

❋ Mother always called just when Loretta was getting to the interesting part of her Kegel routine.

ESSENTIALS

PELVIC FLOOR MUSCLES

A woman's pelvic floor muscles run from the pubic bone at the front to the coccyx or tail bone. During pregnancy, these muscles are given the added job of supporting the womb and the baby. Exercising them regularly during pregnancy will keep them well toned and help lessen the chance of bladder control problems after delivery.

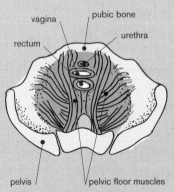

vagina — pubic bone
rectum — urethra
pelvis — pelvic floor muscles

FEMALE PELVIC FLOOR MUSCLES

pelvis

LOCATION OF PELVIS

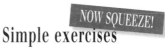

Simple exercises

Here are some simple pelvic floor exercises to try out. Sit, stand, or lie down with your legs slightly apart. Tighten and pull up the muscles around your back passage, and hold them for as long as is comfortable for you, or until the tension begins to fade, and then relax. It's no good trying to hang on when you can feel the tension starting to slip, it doesn't have the same effect. Shorter, stronger holds are what you need. Repeat this at least four times, making sure that you breathe normally, and then repeat the process with the muscles around your vagina and pee hole. Then do a series of four or five quick contractions and releases with each muscle group.

Do these exercises as often as you can, and for as long as you can. You really can't do them often enough. If you find it hard to remember to do them, try to associate them with something you do several times a day, such as making a hot drink or using the telephone, and then do a few exercises every time you switch on the kettle or lift the receiver. A common trick is to do them every time you're standing in line. That's why so many pregnant women sport strange expressions when they're waiting at the checkout.

Another simple way to power up your pelvic floor is to practice tilting or rocking exercises. Put on some loose, comfortable clothing and then lie down on the floor, using as many pillows as it takes to get comfortable. Bend your knees and keep both feet flat on the floor. Put one hand under the small of your back and the other hand flat on your tummy. Tighten the muscles in your tummy and tilt up your butt so that the small of your back is pressed down on your hand. Hold this position for four seconds, breathing normally, and then relax. Repeat five times. Try to do these pelvic tilts at least twice a day: for example, before going to sleep and when you wake up.

EXMERCISE DURING PREGNANCY

The world is divided into those who love to work out, and those who love to work out new reasons to avoid working out. The gym is one of those places that you either love with a passion or will do anything to avoid—a bit like Disney World. If you live in the health club, you might already know the score when it comes to exercise during pregnancy, because you know the difference between a BMI and an IBM (one tells you how many megabites you've had; one tells you how many megabytes you've got left).

If you've never lifted anything heavier than a Gucci purse or a large Manhattan and think that a step class is something to do with salsa lessons or a short-cut to the latest Jimmy Choos, you might be surprised to find your attitude changing over the coming months. Pregnancy often turns confirmed couch potatoes into aspiring Lycra-clad gym junkies: it could be the clean living and the early nights, or it could be the horrible realization that whatever shape your body is in now, various bits are starting to head south and it's about to get a whole lot worse. Your body is changing by the minute, and however fit you are, there are some big differences that must be taken into account.

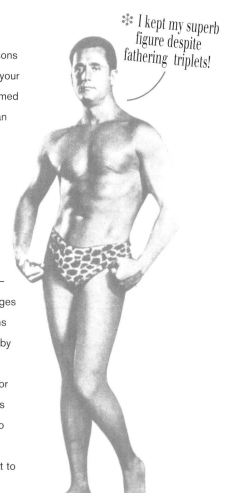

✳ *I kept my superb figure despite fathering triplets!*

Relaxing and relaxin

For starters, there's the stuff called relaxin that we mentioned earlier on—it's a hormone, not a reference to chilling out (*see page 30*), and it changes the game more dramatically than a Tiger Woods tee shot. Relaxin loosens the joints so that there's a bit more give when it comes to getting the baby out, but it doesn't just target the pelvis: it softens up muscles that don't need to be softened up. This means that it's much easier to overstretch or strain other ligaments, joints, and muscles, particularly those in the ankles and knees (which are carrying a heavier load than usual and struggling to handle hormonal clumsiness) and the back (also under pressure from the extra weight, not to mention your shifting center of gravity). So try not to

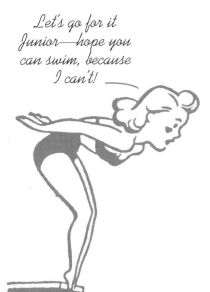

Let's go for it Junior—hope you can swim, because I can't!

IN THE SWIM

Swimming is a perfect pregnancy exercise. It provides an all around cardiac workout and because the weight of your body is supported by the water, there's almost no chance of muscle damage and no chance of impact injury—assuming you don't dive into the shallow end! Swimming strengthens the back muscles, which will reduce backache, and lessens leg edema. If you find it uncomfortable to do breaststroke for any length of time, try using goggles and a snorkle to avoid straining your neck.

overstretch even if you think you can—taking pregnancy yoga and stretch classes is a great way to help prevent overstretching and straining the muscles. Focus on upper body exercises because they are much less likely to divert oxygen from your baby and avoid anything which involves extreme rotation of the spine because there is a very, very, tiny chance that they could pull the placenta away from your womb. Pilates is a no-no in the first 12 weeks, and you should always take advice from a qualified Pilates instructor to devise a program that's suitable for pregnancy. It's probably a better technique to use for shifting and toning post-baby flab.

Extra air

All that stuff about eating for two during pregnancy is complete nonsense, but you are breathing for two when you're pregnant. This explains why you can get more breathless than a B-list starlet doing a passionate love scene. Unless you're really into science, the numbers make as much sense as a bank statement after the Christmas sales. However, the bottom line is that interest rates have just been cut. Your hypothalamus—the bit of your brain that acts like a bank manager—alters deposits and withdrawals in the lungs so that more oxygen goes in and more carbon dioxide comes out. You also get an overdraft facility in the form of the alveoli, tiny little bunches like grapes inside the lungs, which allow gases to pass from the lungs into the bloodstream, and vice versa. This offers a 40 percent increase in transactions, pumping in even more oxygen and expelling even more carbon dioxide.

The breathing rate doesn't alter, but these physical changes make you breathe more deeply. The amount of air exhaled each minute increases by around 50 percent. This makes some women more aware of their breathing and conscious of the need to suck in as much air as possible. Your resting heart rate will probably be a bit higher now that you're pregnant. This doesn't mean you're becoming less fit, it's just that your heart has to pump a great deal more blood around and there's also this little detour called Junior. However, it's important to keep an eye on your heart rate when you're exercising. You can buy little wristwatch monitors in most sports stores. So long as your heart rate doesn't go above 140bpm (beats per minute), your baby will be fine. Anything higher than 140/150 can decrease fetal oxygenation and cause fetal distress.

As you get bigger, your center of gravity shifts, affecting your sense of balance. Take extra care, particularly in changing rooms: wet floors probably cause more damage than workouts! It's also important to wear a good sports bra, and shoes with plenty of support at the ankles and instep. Dehydration is even more dangerous now, so drink plenty of water before and after training. If you leave it until you actually feel thirsty, you'll already be a bit dehydrated. Overheating can also be bad news, so stop if you're starting to feel uncomfortably hot. A quick way to cool down is to run cold water over the veins in your wrists for a few minutes.

What to avoid

Some exercises, like sit ups, are not a good idea, because they can cause the two bands of muscle that run down your belly to separate. This will happen late in pregnancy anyway, but if they split too soon you can end up with funny bulges, like hernias, and this is not a good look. Once you start getting big, you should minimize any floor exercises that involve lying on your back. Apart from the obvious problem of getting up again, you'll block your blood supply by squishing the vena cava (*see also page 94*). If you feel dizzy at any time, stop and lie on your side for a few minutes with your knees bent—it's called the recovery position, but the fetal position is a description that works, too. Weights are OK, so long as they're tiny ones: nothing more than 1 pound (500 g).

❊ My last night at the bowling alley — soon I'll have my very own heavy round object to play with.

Pregnancy isn't a good time to start a tough new workout regime, or take up a new, highly active sport, like squash. However, if you were physically active before conceiving, there's no reason for you to change your routine now. If you have any other risk factors, such as an incompetent cervix, a low lying placenta, or a previous miscarriage, ask your doctor or nurse-midwife for advice. Other conditions that may cause problems include pre-eclampsia, diabetes, and anemia.

Some sports are best avoided. You've probably already worked out that sports with a risk of a high-speed impact such as skydiving, downhill skiing, and car racing are not a good idea (you'd get stuck in the car for starters). Riding, ice-skating, and skiing are out—even experts can take a fall. Cycling is OK until your belly gets so big that your center of gravity starts to shift, increasing the risk of taking a spill (a stationary exercise bike is fine). Waterskiing is also a bad idea because you could get a turbo-charged douche. Similarly, contact sports such as football, kickboxing, and judo are not recommended. Pressure changes and your changing oxygen demands also rule out scuba diving.

No more excuses

Whatever form of exercise you choose, you must learn to listen to your body, and stop when it says it's had enough. You need to get a bit breathless to increase your aerobic strength, but you should never be gasping for air. Keep an eye on the clock: too little exercise is pointless, and too much can do more harm than good. It's not healthy for you to get exhausted, and many of the body chemicals we release during a heavy workout don't suit growing babies. If you weren't particularly active before, a 20–30 minute session is plenty. Aim for three workouts a week to achieve the right balance of work and play and optimum cardiovascular benefits. Alternate between something aerobic—activities that make you a

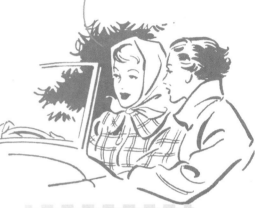

This is what I call getting plenty of fresh air.

AVOID TOP GEAR

Pregnant bodies are a bit like classic cars—they don't like getting overheated. Apart from the fact that you may pass out, getting too hot, particularly during the first trimester, can cause neurological damage to your baby. A gentle glow is fine, a dripping beetroot look isn't. When you are working out, wear loose cotton clothes and if you think you have overdone it, strip off and have a cool shower or run cold water over the bit of your wrists where the veins are visible.

ESSENTIALS

SCHOOL SQUAT

It's amazing how your balance improves — I haven't spilt any tea at all...

If you plan to give birth in the squatting position—and there are good arguments for this because it does mean you get some extra help from gravity—start working on your thigh muscles now. Toddlers may be able to squat for hours, but adult legs quickly get out of the habit. If you don't believe me, time yourself to see how long you can squat without falling over, getting cramps, or your leg muscles turning to jelly. Walking and any exercises that stretch the legs and increase suppleness will help. Another trick is to squat as you watch the TV. If you can make it through an episode of *ER*, you're doing really well.

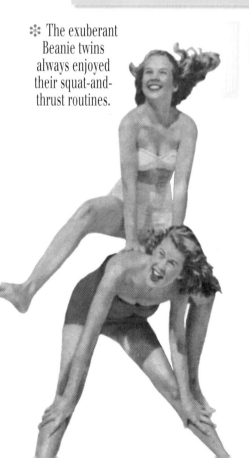

❉ The exuberant Beanie twins always enjoyed their squat-and-thrust routines.

bit out of breath—and something stretchy and gentle, like yoga. Set realistic targets and try to incorporate exercises you enjoy. If it's just a hassle, you'll find excuses for not doing it. If you're taking a class or getting advice from a trainer, make sure that he or she really knows his or her stuff. Some trainers are well informed in general, but haven't got a clue about the extra risks involved in being a mom-to-be. Ask to see the trainer's certificates, and find out how much insurance the gym has. Questions of this kind should focus the manager's mind nicely.

Workouts that work

If you've been a slouch on the couch too long and you want to get into better shape, there are plenty of soft options that are perfect for pregnancy, including walking, swimming, and yoga. Anything that strengthens the back will delay the onset of backache (there's no avoiding it completely), and reduce the risk of long-term postural problems. Activities that strengthen the tummy muscles will give you a bit more oomph when it comes to pushing, as well as helping your abdominals spring back into shape. (Well, they may stroll back rather than spring back, but every little bit helps.)

ANKLE CIRCLES

Pregnancy hormones make the veins more stretchy, which is why you might get cramps, varicose veins, and swollen ankles. A simple exercise for improving the circulation is to circle each foot at the ankle, starting with 12 turns in each direction. You can do this sitting or lying down, but make sure that your legs are properly supported: you're asking for trouble if you try to do any sort of leg lift when you're flat on your back.

Let's turn the spare room into a gym, darling — nurseries are so last year.

Walking (and we mean stepping out at a brisk pace, not dawdling down the shopping mall) provides a great low-impact aerobic workout, not to mention some much needed time-out from the world. Aim to be just a little bit breathless: if you've got so little puff that you can't talk, then you're overdoing it. If in doubt, you can talk to yourself, reciting all those things that you're meant to do during the day but will probably forget. Remember to take a water bottle. Unless you train regularly and really know what you're doing, don't go jogging, because it inflicts a bigger shakeup than a corporate takeover, and puts a lot of pressure on the pelvic floor. If you're a well-conditioned athlete and you're determined to continue, then carry on jogging, but listen to your body and don't push yourself past comfort.

Swimming is a superb exercise to do during pregnancy (*see page 103*) but don't dive or jump into the water, use the steps or sit at the side of the pool and slip in gently. Never rush when you're in the changing rooms or walking to and from the pool—your changing center of gravity means that you're already pretty clumsy and wet floors add to the risk of a slip or fall. Dancing can be an enjoyable way of working out, too. In a lot of cultures, moms-to-be are taught their own special moves: in fact, belly-dancing got started this way, working on the "If you've got it, flaunt it" principle. Circling the hips and doing little rhythmic tilts can help to relieve backache and muscular tension in the small of the back. If nothing else, it will provide a few laughs. The mixture of gentle stretches, focused breathing, and relaxation techniques to be found in yoga covers all the bases brilliantly. If you practice the relaxation bits, you might become able to consciously lower your blood pressure. This might not sound like much of a party trick right now, but if your blood pressure becomes too high later on (*see pages 76–77*), it could keep you out of the hospital.

WEIGHING UP

The idea of eating for two went completely out of the window at around the same time that women got the vote, so tempting as it may be, don't kid yourself that pregnancy is the perfect excuse to cut loose with the cookie jar. And it's definitely not the time to try to restrict your weight gain either, because babies benefit from a few wobbly bits and any diet that's restrictive is probably restricting the flow of nutrients that's reaching your baby.

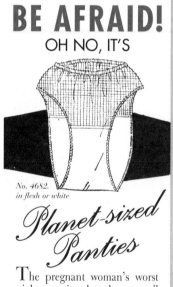

BE AFRAID!
OH NO, IT'S

No. 4682.
in flesh or white

Planet-sized Panties

The pregnant woman's worst nightmare is what doctors call *Maximus pantius.* Act now to protect yourself by sending for our discreetly wrapped brochure.

No. 2586.
French knicker, in floral canvas. Doubles as shower cap. Available in Large, Ex-Large, Huge, Mammoth, and Godzilla.

Vegetarians, vegans, and women with lactose intolerance really need to do their homework and watch that they're not missing anything important. In the 1980s, British researchers came across detailed records for 1,600 babies born between 1911 and 1930, and found that size really does matter. When these babies, now adults, were tracked down, some spooky patterns began to emerge. Fullterm babies who had weighed less than 5 pounds (2.5 kg) at birth had twice the average rate of heart disease, and were much more likely to get diabetes. The heavyweight babies who were born with a bit of extra bounce, or acquired some before their first birthday, also fared poorly.

So what should you aim for? The recommended average weight gain range is between 25 and 35 pounds (11–16 kg), depending on your BMI. To calculate your BMI, divide your weight in kilograms by the square of your height in meters. For example, a woman who weighs 70 kg (154 pounds) and is 1.7 meters (5 feet, six inches) tall has a BMI of 24 (70 divided by 2.89). Many nutrition web sites have BMI calculators in English and metric if you don't want to do the math yourself! Even if you lose weight in the first trimester because of nausea, some data supports that this can cause the placenta to compensate with increased growth and results in even bigger babies.

As a rule of thumb (or bum), your weight gain should be slow and steady in the early weeks: around 3 or 4 pounds (about 2 kg) in the first trimester if you want to avoid a lecture from your doctor. It should then pick up to about 1 pound (500 g) a week for the rest of the pregnancy, although it often tails off toward the end. This is a rough guide, because any number of things can affect the process. If you have bad morning sickness and spend the first trimester with your head down the john, you might lose weight, or only put on a teenie amount. A surge in the final weeks could be a sign of pre-eclampsia, a really serious Häagen Dazs habit, or even a change of scales. (Check that any dips and peaks are not just a matter of discrepancies between different scales and weighing machines.) It also depends on where you're coming from. If you were Calista Flockhart-skinny to start with, you'll have some ground to make up and could put on 44 pounds (20 kg) or more. If you've got more curves than a Chesterfield, you probably need only a little extra upholstery.

✳ Great! I'm all prepared for tonight's dinner. Now I'd better go shopping for tomorrow's supplies.

Genetic clues

If you've got good hunter-gatherer genes (and we're not talking about the summer sales), you'll have to watch your weight more carefully. For clues, check out the women in your family who've already had kids. Some women are biologically programmed to stack on as much weight as possible during pregnancy. This was great when we were all scrabbling around in the savannah, not knowing where our next pile of nuts and berries was coming from, because the saddlebags on our butts and thighs could provide plenty of reserves to keep the breastmilk flowing. Back then, a big butt was a sign of beauty and awesome childrearing ability. In some cultures, it still is: have you ever seen a fertility goddess who looked like Sarah Jessica Parker?

HOW IT ADDS UP

To keep tabs on how much weight you are gaining, it's a good idea to start a food journal and note down everything that you eat and drink. You might be eating like a bird, but honey, are we talking sparrow or ostrich? If you are at the trough more frequently than Miss Piggy, a journal will reveal the awful truth. It will also provide you and your physician with a few clues about where to cut back, and which nutrients you might be missing out on.

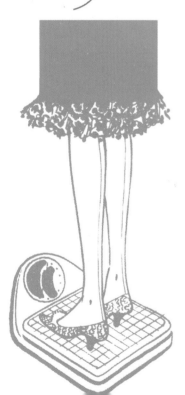

✳ Who would have thought that Manolos and Moschino could weigh so very much?

If you are gaining weight too quickly or too slowly, your physician may want to run a few extra tests just to make sure that everything's OK. Roughly speaking, your baby makes up about one-fourth of the weight you'll gain, around 7½ pounds (2.9 kg). At least another fourth is made up of the fat stores that are needed for breast-feeding. The rest covers all the extras and equipment that is needed to keep things ticking over. Extra bulk in the uterus adds around 2 pounds (900 g), the placenta is around 1½ pounds (680 g), and the amniotic fluid can be anything from 1 to 2 pounds (450–900 g), depending how much there is. Bigger boobies add another pound or so (around 450 g), and the extra blood needed to service this lot weighs around 4 pounds (1.8 kg).

Sound bites

Energy needs to increase by around 200 calories a day during pregnancy, but all calories are not created equal, so it makes sense to think in terms of quality, not quantity. Many of us eat so poorly that we get more calories than we need and still fall short of a lot of dietary goals. Healthful eating is a lot simpler than it might seem: you don't have to be a domestic goddess to make the grade. The trick is to eat high-quality food that is fresh enough to remember where it came from, and hasn't had a lot of its nutrients processed to death. Another good number to remember is five. Everyone, pregnant or not, should eat five servings of fruit and vegetables every day.

This reduces your odds of getting heart disease and cancer, and fills you up with so much good stuff that you'll struggle to squeeze in the bad stuff. There's also a lot of sense to the old wives' tale that you should get a mix of colors, which is a simple way to get a range of vitamins and disease-busting antioxidants. One serving is the equivalent of an apple or banana, or a cup of smaller fruit, dried fruit, or vegetables. Potatoes don't count—they're classified as carbohydrates—so don't kid yourself that you can fill your quota by ordering fries with everything. Juice counts as only one serving, even if you drink a lot of it.

No exclusions

Exclusion diets of any kind need serious thought. In some circles, food fads and bizarre eating plans have become a must-have accessory to rank along with a Prada purse. During pregnancy, though, most of them are unnecessary, unhealthy, and unwise. Very few of the people who claim to have a food allergy or intolerance actually have one. Get your facts right first and ask your doctor for a credible test, and don't exclude any foods without medical advice.

Going vegetarian or vegan may be a life choice for you, but it's one that needs a lot of caution, care, and commitment if you're going to impose it on a growing baby. Plant sources of protein don't contain the full complement of amino acids; to ensure you get the full range, they have to be combined with dairy products, or wheat and other grains. Other good stuff, like zinc and iron, tends to be associated with animal proteins, too. Good sources of plant proteins include legumes (such as beans, peas, and lentils), meat substitutes (such as Quorn and tofu), soy, nuts, grains, seeds, mushrooms, peas, and brewer's yeast.

If you don't want to go organic, make sure you wash fruit and vegetables thoroughly. A squirt of dishwashing liquid added to the water will cut through waxy chemicals and residues.

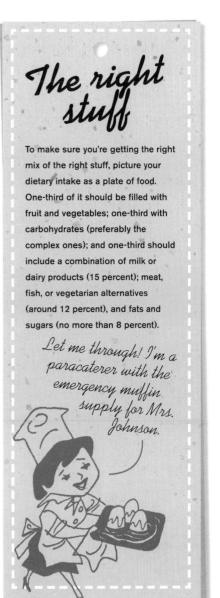

The right stuff

To make sure you're getting the right mix of the right stuff, picture your dietary intake as a plate of food. One-third of it should be filled with fruit and vegetables; one-third with carbohydrates (preferably the complex ones); and one-third should include a combination of milk or dairy products (15 percent); meat, fish, or vegetarian alternatives (around 12 percent), and fats and sugars (no more than 8 percent).

Let me through! I'm a paracaterer with the emergency muffin supply for Mrs. Johnson.

GOOD TASTE OR A BAD TASTE?

If you thought that pregnancy could do some wacky things to your sexual appetite, it's nothing compared to what it does to your tastebuds and to your appetite, or not, for food. And just when you think you've come up with an eating plan that provides plenty of nourishment while bypassing problems such as nausea and indigestion, your pregnancy hormones go through a gear change and it's back to the drawing board, or cutting board, once again.

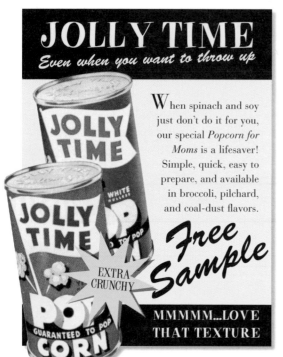

There are a lot of different reasons for these changes. For starters—and we're not talking appetizers here—there's morning sickness and cravings, and then there's the way that pregnancy hormones change your sense of smell. This isn't just a matter of triggering aversions to certain foods—although there's no denying that it does; it also changes the taste of food. Sounds crazy? It's not. The broad brushstrokes of sweet, sour, and salty are firmly tied to the tastebuds on our tongues, but a lot of the subtle strokes that fill in the finer details of our sense of taste come from aromas and the way that they waft past certain sensors in our nasal passages. Pregnancy alters our sense of smell, and along with it our sense of taste. Karen, a 31-year-old first-timer who works in the catering trade, says, "We do a great deal of corporate entertaining—you know, up-market nibbles, little pastries, and so on. Normally it's a struggle not to grab a snack when I'm talking to the chefs, but for the first couple of months of my pregnancy I couldn't set foot in the kitchens. The smell of food frying was the worst, it went straight to my stomach."

It's not the only thing that changes. Texture can suddenly become important—although moms are more likely to talk about this one than scientists. There's not a lot in the way of research on the subject—other than the consumption figures for such orally

❄ Thank goodness Gloria had taken the Comfort Food Course at the Doris Day Institute.

KEEP IT LIGHT

Aim for three light meals a day, plus a couple of snacks (apples, nuts, high-protein bars, or dried fruit, not Oreos and ice cream). But if nausea, heartburn, and the baby pushing up into your stomach are killing your appetite, eat a series of smaller meals and snacks instead.

textural experiences as chips, popcorn, and ice cream—but ask any mom in the making, or mom of young children, and they'll tell you that factors like crunchiness or smoothness are all-important. Not convinced? Think of milk chocolate and the chances are, you think in terms of texture. The downside of this is that when you're pregnant certain textures—for some reason, they're often the ones attached to green vegetables—may suddenly seem slimy and extremely unpleasant.

For most of the time that you're pregnant, you'll probably be happier grazing and snacking than sitting down to a Thanksgiving-style pig-out—or should that be turkey-out? Again, the reasons vary. In the early days, it's largely down to morning sickness and being too tired to cook. As your bulge begins to really bulge, it's more to do with shrinking stomach space, expanding baby, and the pain of heartburn. "At first, I found the whole food thing really difficult," says Jessica, who works in PR and often had to take clients out to long lunches. "Then I realized that what I really wanted was a couple of appetizers and a dessert. To be honest, some days I probably wanted an appetizer and two desserts, but I didn't think that was such a good idea. If I was with someone who really liked their food, I'd order a side salad as well—it made them feel more comfortable without making me feel really uncomfortable."

Preparation time is a factor, too. When you're hungry, you want food, and you want it fast—but that doesn't have to mean you have to resort to junk food. Not many meals are quicker than a poached egg, an avocado with shrimp, or steamed asparagus with a shaving of Parmesan. Broiled chicken or fish can be given a complete makeover with a sprinkling of herbs, ginger, or lemon juice. Experiment with salsas: try diced strawberries, cucumber, and freshly ground pepper; or chopped oranges, tomatoes, and scallions. Light soups go down well, and can be made in advance and frozen. Boston beans on toast beats a burger hands down.

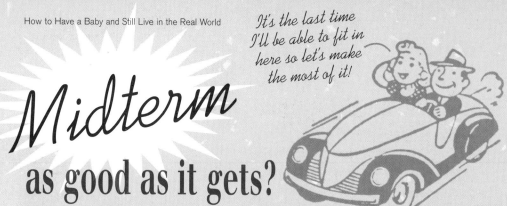

It's the last time I'll be able to fit in here so let's make the most of it!

Midterm
as good as it gets?

Bkaby, you've never had it so good. Once you make it into the second trimester, things start to look up: you're past all the nailbiting tests and scans; everyone knows the news; your partner has stopped wearing his stunned mullet look; his mother has realized that there's no point offering advice; and you and your partner are finally getting your heads around the concept of parenthood.

✳ The triplets slowly realized that the moment for Dutch caps had passed.

Then there are the physical changes. Hormone surges stabilize, and usually take morning sickness with them. If you're going to "bloom," this is when it will happen. However, don't take it for granted. For some women, pregnancy is a matter of gritty urban realism rather than gardening metaphors.

Face facts

If you're a bloomer, the changes in your skin condition might knock off more years than a face-lift. Some of this is down to your newfound healthy lifestyle, and extra hormones mean that everything works overtime, including the natural oils that moisturize the skin. Your extra blood supply adds roses to your cheeks, while the extra fluid pushes out wrinkles better than collagen shots. That's the upside. The downside is that when the extra sweat mixes with all that extra oil and body heat, your skin could end up looking like a pepperoni pizza—check with your healthcare provider about which products are safer to use. You might even acquire skin tags—little bobbles of skin and fat that pop out in the strangest places. Most of them go away in time, but it's not guaranteed.

GONE LATER

Hair today

Your hair changes too, and will get more bounce than a bankrupt's checkbook. It doesn't grow more quickly, but the hormonal changes make it hang on for longer, so you get more volume. (The effect is reversed once you give birth, and it will come out in handfuls. This is only temporary because you're just losing nine or ten months' worth in one or two months.) The extra oils will make it shine more, although it may need to be washed more often.

Pregnancy hormones mean that you might also react differently to hair dyes. Some doctors get very twitchy about using hair color products during pregnancy, although there's not a lot of evidence either way regarding birth defects. Highlighting with silver foils away from the roots is fine. If you're unlucky enough to be going gray, use natural vegetable dyes such as henna, and always do the skin and strand tests suggested on the package.

During the midterm months, those soft-focus photos of pregnant women looking wistful and dreamy might start to make a tiny bit of sense. Don't be surprised if you find yourself patting your bump, covering it protectively when you're caught in a crowd, or asking it whether it prefers tuna or chicken for supper. A lot of this behavior is instinctive, but there's a lot to be said for taking time out each day to relax and focus on your baby. In traditional Chinese medicine, it's called tai-kyo, and stems from the belief that the mother's mood during pregnancy can affect the health of her child. Mood-altering body chemicals like adrenaline and endorphins cross the placenta, so it makes medical sense, too.

Bumpsie can hear what's going on from about five months, and will learn to recognize your voice and other familiar sounds before the birth. Some mothers are so keen (or so crazy, depending on your view of these things) that they schedule in regular sessions of foreign languages, Rachmaninov recitals, and talking books. Personally, I figured I was doing well if I remembered my antenatal appointments.

✳ Well, sugar pie, I'll do my very best to help you out.

✳ Oh Chuck, my hair looks so gorgeous, I want to be pregnant all the time!

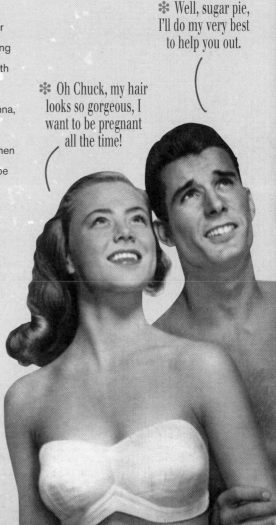

BACK TO SCHOOL PRENATAL CLASSES

Prenatal classes, also called antenatal or parentcraft classes or birthing or childbirth education, can never completely prepare you for labor; only a previous delivery can do that, and even then there are no gilt-edged guarantees. However, knowledge is power, and it will give you a degree of control when push comes to push. Classes are now such an everyday part of pregnancy that it's hard to imagine what it must have been like—and it wasn't that long ago—when women went into labor without any real knowledge about what was going to happen.

I've read through *Little Women* twice, and there's absolutely no mention of eating your placenta.

A good prenatal class is a bit like a good buffet: you might not fancy the smoked salmon, but it's nice to know it's there if you do. Classes should point out all the issues and provide a working knowledge of what can happen, what can go wrong, and your options at every turn. Bad classes lay down dogmatic rules, set unrealistic expectations, and generally make you feel lousy if you don't toe the line. Don't be bullied into believing there is a "right" way: there isn't, and some of the best prenatal classes pinch ideas from different approaches. Another mistake is to think that you don't need classes if you're having a C-section. Classes cover a lot more than the delivery itself, and provide a great chance to swap notes with other moms-to-be. The trick is to find the one that best suits you and your partner. Get it right, and you'll probably forge friendships that last a lifetime; get it wrong, and you'll get some early practice in stress control and pain management.

Brainpower

Back in the 1930s, an Englishman called Grantly Dick-Read (seriously, that was his name) formulated the theory that the fear of the unknown caused muscle tension, which made labor more painful. The more painful things got, the more frightened and tense the woman became. He argued that this vicious cycle could be broken if women knew what to expect, and learned a few basic relaxation techniques to provide a distraction from contractions. Nowadays it's called the psychophysical approach—which is really just a fancy way of saying "keep your cool"—and his ideas seem so blindingly obvious that it's hard to believe that he was written off as a crackpot for many years. Another wacky Dick-Read idea that took a long time to catch on was that it was better to leave the baby with mom rather than rushing it off to a bright, terrifyingly sterile nursery. Not until the 1950s did classes based on Dick-Read's ideas (also known as the Gamper method after a nurse-midwife he worked with) become widely accepted.

Lamaze

The next big breakthrough came courtesy of some mouthwatering Russian dogs. Sounds screwy? It's perfectly true. By giving dogs food every time a bell rang, the Nobel-prizewinning Russian physiologist Ivan Pavlov trained them to cut out the middle man and salivate whenever they heard the sound of the bell. He called it conditioning, and a French doctor called Fernand Lamaze figured out that the same techniques could be used to control pain during labor. The Lamaze method has become the most popular method in the USA, and forms the basis of NCT (National Childbirth Trust) classes in Britain.

It takes commitment and plenty of practice, but the basic idea is that you learn breathing patterns and exercises that condition your body to work with the contractions, rather than against them. Your birth partner is an important part of the process, and acts as a breathing coach, watching the run of play and knowing when to suggest a different breathing pattern. Lamaze works if you do. The more you practice, the more antipain points you have in the bank. If you skip classes and forget to do your homework, you could find that there's nothing to draw on when the big day comes.

FIND A CLASS ACT

A good starting point is to ask your nurse-midwife or physician whether there are any classes that they particularly recommend. They will know what's available locally and how they fit with their own personal styles. Sure, it's all about what you want, but it does save a lot of time and tension if your carer and classes follow roughly the same script. There's no point in signing up for the earth mother special before booking a C-section and stocking up on feeding bottles. Work out roughly what you want in pregnancy, labor, and parenthood, and look for classes that aim for the same things.

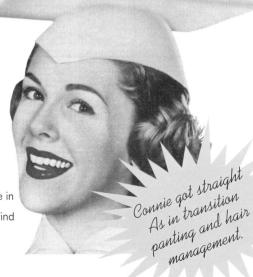

Connie got straight As in transition panting and hair management.

Bradley method

Dr. Robert A. Bradley pioneered the natural birth movement in the USA with the American Academy of Husband-Coached Childbirth. Drugs of any kind are discouraged during labor and breast-feeding (it's assumed that you will breast-feed), and you are encouraged to "tune in" to your body and take control of labor. Breathing techniques are important, but unlike Lamaze it's all about long, deep, controlled breaths, rather than a mixture of deep breathing and panting like Sharon Stone in *Basic Instinct*. School sometimes starts early with the Bradley method, because it includes a lot of work on using good nutrition to prevent problems. A typical course will run for 12 weeks, starting in month five or six. If you're keen on the idea of a drug-free delivery, the success rate is good: more than 90 percent of Bradley graduates give birth without medication.

French connections OOH LA LA!

More recently, French obstetricians Frederick LeBoyer and Michel Odent have pushed—sorry, encouraged us to push—for a more baby-centered, natural approach. LeBoyer argues that babies are incredibly sensitive to external influences, and that their primal needs for warmth and comfort are overshadowed by the bright lights and bustle of delivery rooms. There is very little evidence to support his theories, but they sound reasonable enough—well, they do until he loses the plot and suggests that the mother is the "enemy" of her baby, forcing him or her out of the womb and crushing him or her within the birth canal. It's a guilt trip that most women can do without, which is why most classes don't preach "pure" LeBoyer. On the plus side, LeBoyer stresses the importance of bonding, something that mothers have always instinctively understood, but doctors didn't stumble upon until recently. LeBoyer babies are delivered directly onto the mom's tummy, left to enjoy a cuddle, and offered the breast soon after birth.

THE DARK AGES

Ignorance isn't bliss: try to imagine how you would feel if your contractions started, and all you knew was that it was going to hurt like hell, it could last a long time, and you might die in the process? It's hardly surprising that women used to die in childbirth. It wasn't until the late 18th century and early 19th century that people like Alexander Gordon in Britain, and Oliver Wendell Holmes in the United States, made the connection between poor hygiene and postpartum blood poisoning. Not long afterward, a Viennese doctor came up with a brilliant new technique that dramatically reduced death rates. His big idea? "Hey guys, why don't we wash our hands first!"

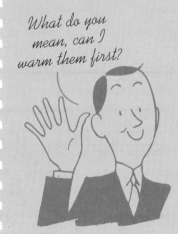

What do you mean, can I warm them first?

Michel Odent argues that women should throw their inhibitions out of the window and follow their natural instincts. He suggests turning down the lights, putting on relaxing music, and trying to make the whole thing as gentle and stressfree as possible. He also argues that painkillers and analgesics are counterproductive, because they short-circuit the endorphins that provide natural pain relief. It's not as wacky as it sounds. The sensation of pain kick-starts the production of endorphins, and levels gradually build up as contractions get stronger. Odent was one of the first childbirth gurus to encourage women to try different birthing positions: on all fours, squatting, even hanging from a chandelier if it seems like a good idea. He was also the first to use birthing pools. He thought that they would help with pain relief, and when the women didn't want to get out, he delivered babies into the water. Babies are under water in the womb, so there's no danger of them drowning. It's not until they hit the air that they breathe in and use their lungs.

Best of the rest

Sheila Kitzinger takes the view that childbirth should be an empowering and life-altering experience. It can be, and there's a lot to be said for her no-nonsense, earthy style, but ask a woman who's been in labor for 24 hours what she thinks about the beauty of childbirth, and she might feel empowered to deliver a stiff uppercut or a sharp kick to the shins.

Health-maintenance organizations, hospitals, and groups such as the International Childbirth Education Association all offer prenatal classes that borrow bits from all over the place. The advantage of this scattergun approach is that you cover all the bases and learn a little bit about every philosophy, which makes it easier to go with the flow once the action starts. This is particularly important the first time around, when you really don't know how your mind and body will handle the whole thing.

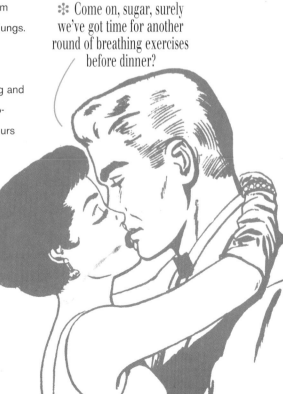

❋ Come on, sugar, surely we've got time for another round of breathing exercises before dinner?

THE BEST-LAID PLANS...

Now's the time to while away a few hours making plans: win the lottery, wow Steven Spielberg with an idea for a screenplay, learn how to spot an Old Master at a garage sale...oh, and then there's your birth plan. A birth plan is a great way to prepare for labor, so long as you're not silly enough to think that things are going to play out exactly as you want them to, because they rarely do. As Woody Allen said, "If you want to make God laugh, tell him about your plans."

Like designer baby accessories, birth plans are a relatively recent phenomenon. They have no legal status, and some doctors and nurse-midwives treat them as a bit of a joke. If you'd seen a few hundred of them, you'd understand why. Trust me, you've got a better chance of being taken seriously if you skip the playlist of pet sounds that you want on the music system, and your request for industrial quantities of Chanel No. 5 throughout.

Prima gravida or prima donna?

Follow your mom's time-honored advice: ask nicely, and use phrases like "I would prefer" and "if possible," rather than, "If I don't get my epidural the minute I ask for it, I'll sue you into oblivion, dog breath!" Stick to the basics, and show that you know the difference between a prima gravida and a prima donna. In some cases it's a fine line, and you'll get the best out of the medical staff if you don't cross it. It's OK to use medical terms and abbreviations, but make sure you've got the right ones. An IV isn't your inner voice, and requesting a VBAC won't get you a very big armchair (for the record, they're an intravenous line and a vaginal birth after a Cesarean, respectively). Keep your birth plan brief and crystal clear. If your baby's in distress and you're screaming so loudly that the people in the geriatric ward are complaining, your obstetrician probably won't feel inclined to read 10,000 carefully chosen words on your idea of an ideal birth. The whole point about birth plans is that they aren't about perfection, and half the time

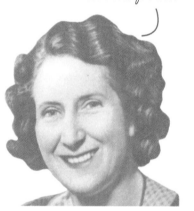

Pretty please with sugar on top worked for me.

SIBLING RIVALRY

If you're a second- or third-timer, the most important plan is how to lay your hands on the "must-have" toy of the season required to head off sibling rivalry. But a few years down the line, your goal item will date you more unforgivingly than any passport photo.

they're not even about planning. Setting your thoughts down on paper gives you the chance to ask questions you might not have thought of asking before, and to make alternative arrangements if you don't like the answers. A plan also puts the medics on notice that you've done your homework, and will do your best to make the whole thing as simple and painless as possible. Hopefully, this will encourage them to do the same.

The three Ps

Birth plans are really about the three Ps: possibilities, probabilities, and hospital policies. How long past your due date will you be allowed to go before you're induced? Does the hospital administer enemas and pubic shaves as a matter of routine? If you thought that this stuff only survived in the pages of *Penthouse*, think again. Until recently you wouldn't have had much say in the matter—other than "Ouch!" The theory was that having a pile of poop in your system could block your baby's exit, lead to cross-contamination or unbearable embarrassment. Enemas are almost unheard of today—there's nothing like labor contractions to cause you to offload your load; there's more chance of cross-contamination with an enema; and embarrassment isn't really an issue when you're screaming like a fishwife, ripping off your clothes because you're too hot, and calling the love of your life an uncaring asshole.

✳ I love the part where you demand world peace and live whale song.

Ideally, you should have covered a lot of this territory when you decided on the type of maternity care you wanted. Are you an earth mother or a mommy's girl? Are you a health diva or a health disaster? Is pain part of the process, or something that should only accompany credit card statements, fashionable shoes, and visits to the dentist?

Here are some questions that are worth considering: who do you want in the delivery room? Are friends, older children, and personal gurus allowed? (And do you really want them there?) Do you want to use a TENS machine (*see page 126*)? If so, will there be one available at the hospital or should you rent your own? And will there be someone to help you put it on? How much can you personalize your room? Are you allowed to take drinks and snacks into the delivery room? (Eating a little dried fruit, or sucking on a glucose sweet can provide a much-needed shot of energy, but some hospitals have very strict no-food policies.) Are still and video cameras allowed (personally, we'd ban them)? Will you be hooked up to an IV line like an extra in *ER*? If you want an epidural, will somebody be there to do it right away? Can you get a "mobile" epidural, which will enable you to go walking during labor? After the birth, how long will they let you go without a pee before wanting to put in a catheter? Can you wear contact lenses? (If you need a general anesthetic you can't, but you wouldn't be able to see anything then anyway.) Will you be asked to stay in bed throughout the labor? Can you call the shots on different positions, or will they want to strap you into stirrups like the Bride of Frankenstein? What steps, if any, will be taken to avoid an episiotomy? Will your obstetrician let you tear? Will the baby be delivered directly on to your belly, or whisked off for weighing and a wipe down? Can the father cut the umbilical cord (and does he really want to)? Do you want your baby to be given vitamin K? If so, will this be given by injection or orally? Vitamin K reduces the risk of bleeding but there has been some very scary, but very inconclusive, research linking injections to later problems. Like a lot of pregnancy and childrearing questions, this one has to be your call.

Miriam, who's been there and done the delivery thing three times, admits: "I can be a bit of a control freak, so when I was having my first baby I wrote everything down in my birth plan—and I mean everything. It was a

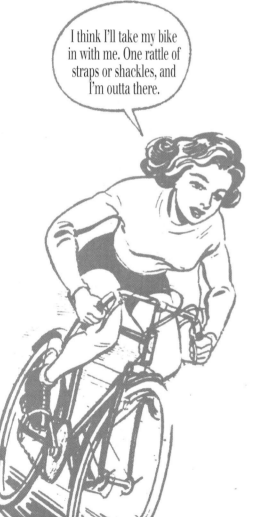

I think I'll take my bike in with me. One rattle of straps or shackles, and I'm outta there.

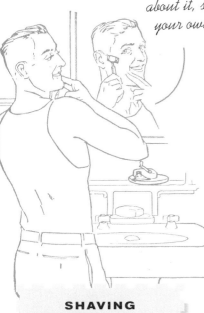

Don't even think about it, sister; get your own razor!

moral and medical maze, with all sorts of statements like, 'If A happens, I want you to do B or C; but if D happens, I want you to do E or F.' There were so many 'if this happens' I don't think they had a clue what I really wanted. Second time around, it was much simpler: 'No C-section! No episiotomy! No catheter!' Third time around, I didn't bother."

Jodie, a 37-year-old second timer, says, "I was really proud of my birth plan. There'd been a few complications during the pregnancy, so I had to cover a lot of possibilities. In the end, everything went by the book, and so quickly that the obstetrician didn't have a chance to read my plan until Julia had been born."

"Use a pencil when you're writing your birth plan," advises Madeleine, 24. "My birth plan was actually part of my notes, so I couldn't just write it out on a new piece of paper. I kept thinking of new things to add, or little bits I wanted to add or take out, but because I'd started writing it in pen I had to use correction fluid to make changes. The sheet was as rigid as cardboard by the end of it all."

SHAVING

Back in the dark ages of gynecology, the theory was that shaving a pregnant woman's pubic hair made everything nice and clean, and germ-free, but there is a lot of evidence that it actually increases the risk of infection through shaving nicks. In some cultures, women prefer to be hair-free. There are very few doctors or nurse-midwives who would advocate this, but if you come across any who are stuck in a timewarp, vote with your feet (and follicles) and find another one. If you care to bare, a depilatory cream is the best bet.

Stat's it

Try to acquire the mindset of one of those baseball nerds who collects stats and facts, because these will give you a lot more useful information than bland statements. For instance, the line "Our episiotomy rate is in line with other birth centers" doesn't mean that you won't get one. In some hospitals, between 80 and 90 percent of first-timers with headfirst deliveries do. Once you get started, you'll probably come up with more questions than a whole season of *Who Wants To Be A Millionaire?* Make sure you've got all the answers before the action starts, because once it does, there'll be no time to phone a friend, there probably won't be an audience to ask (we'll assume you didn't go for the webcam), and you're way past the point of going 50–50.

IT'S A PAIN IN THE ... AAAAARRRRGH!

Until you're actually in labor, you won't know how tough or easy (relatively, that is) it's going to be, so there's no point making too many decisions about pain relief in advance. There are any number of variables, such as the size of your baby, the size of your pelvis, the length of the labor, and the level of support and encouragement you get, which can affect your pain threshold. However, it doesn't hurt (groan!) to arm yourself with all the facts about pain relief in advance.

❊ Dolores had never given a damn, but childbirth was about to change that.

A number of studies have proven that a lot depends on the individual's attitude (the real thing, not the stuff you need for street cred). If you're reasonably confident that you'll cope with the pain, you probably will. It also helps if you really don't give a damn: women who are fearful of letting go or making a complete show of themselves are much more likely to have a tough time. Why the heck should you hold back? If there was ever a time for really letting rip, then this is it. Don't kid yourself that it's not going to hurt, because it will, but so do a lot of other things that are worth having, like stiletto heels, a flat stomach, and good teeth. It's not like the movies, either. For starters, what on earth did they do with all that hot water? Ordinary vaginal deliveries, featuring women who are *not* screaming like Fay Wray in *King Kong*, are the norm, but this makes for deadly dull drama, so we only see screaming gals on television or at the movies. Several studies have shown that women who expect it to hurt, but who are pretty confident that they will cope, report less pain than those who panic and start doubting themselves. Think about it: if labor pains were really that unbearable, no woman would have more than one child.

Try to keep your options open. Don't set yourself unrealistic goals, because you'll simply be laying the groundwork for massive guilt trips. There's nothing wrong with aiming for a drugfree delivery, but don't be afraid to ask for help if you need it. You wouldn't refuse painkillers at the dentist, so why should you refuse them in labor? It's all about pushing out a healthy baby, not proving that you could be Miss August in *Masochism Monthly*. There are no gold medals for going cold turkey, and if you're feeling really bruised and battered by labor, you might miss the magical first moments, or even hours, of your baby's introduction to the world. You'll cope with labor pains much better if you're relaxed, confident, have a pretty good idea of what to expect, know pain relief is there if you want it, and have had some sleep. You're much more likely to start fraying at the edges if you're anxious, tense, tired, worried that you won't cope, hungry or thirsty, left on your own, and have a rigid view of what will happen.

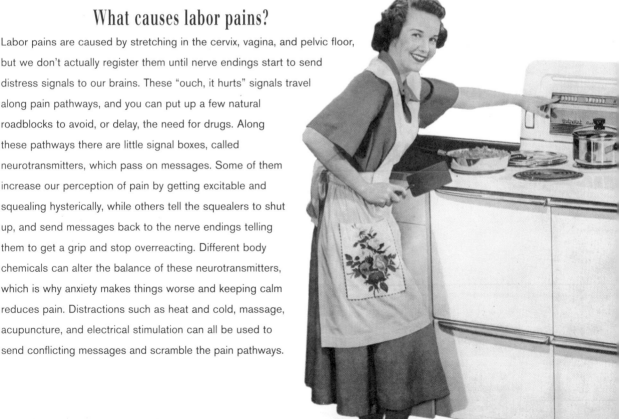

✳ Hetty found that hearty meals always helped fathers-to-be to cope with the early stages of labor.

What causes labor pains?

Labor pains are caused by stretching in the cervix, vagina, and pelvic floor, but we don't actually register them until nerve endings start to send distress signals to our brains. These "ouch, it hurts" signals travel along pain pathways, and you can put up a few natural roadblocks to avoid, or delay, the need for drugs. Along these pathways there are little signal boxes, called neurotransmitters, which pass on messages. Some of them increase our perception of pain by getting excitable and squealing hysterically, while others tell the squealers to shut up, and send messages back to the nerve endings telling them to get a grip and stop overreacting. Different body chemicals can alter the balance of these neurotransmitters, which is why anxiety makes things worse and keeping calm reduces pain. Distractions such as heat and cold, massage, acupuncture, and electrical stimulation can all be used to send conflicting messages and scramble the pain pathways.

SHOCK THERAPY

TENS

TENS (transcutaneous electrical nerve stimulation) is a brilliant roadblock for some women, but is pretty much useless for others. The machine consists of four sets of electrodes. These are stuck to your back and hooked up to a small unit, about the size of a Walkman, which sends out tiny electric shocks. The unit has two controls: one to govern the intensity of the signal, and one to switch the signal on and off. Some hospitals and birth centers provide TENS units, but you can also rent them (make sure the unit is delivered at least two weeks before your due date).

TENS works best when you put it on early and allow for a gradual buildup. On a scale of one to ten, when you first put it on you'll probably find anything over a two or three uncomfortable, but by the end of the labor you'll have it on ten. The big plus of TENS is that the handset puts you in control. The only real downside is that you can't wear it in a shower or a birthing pool.

Pins and needles

Acupuncture works along the same lines as TENS, by releasing natural painkilling endorphins. Be sure to check hospital policy though, some won't allow alternative practitioners anywhere near the labor suite. Acupuncture seems to be most effective among women who've used it before—in part this is probably a placebo effect of previous positive experiences boosting the impact of the treatment.

In a trance

Hypnotherapy has gathered a bad reputation because of showmen in shiny suits, who convince gormless audience volunteers that they are chickens or dogs, or that it would be a laugh to simulate sex with a

ESSENTIALS

LABOR PAINS

Labor pains occur due to stretching and expanding in the cervix, pelvic floor, and vagina. At the same time, the uterus contracts to push the baby out. As the baby makes its way down the birth canal, this adds extra pressure on the spine and pubic bone, and rectum.

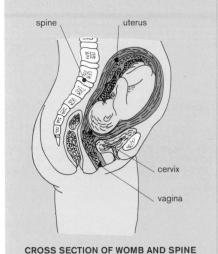

CROSS SECTION OF WOMB AND SPINE

complete stranger. This is a pity, because some women in labor swear by it. Forget all the cornball stuff about gazing into someone's eyes and losing your self-control: that happens only in cheap romantic novels. You can't be hypnotized unless you want to be, and you probably won't even go into a trance (three out of four adults make such lousy subjects that they can't be hypnotized at all). If you want to give it a try, start as soon as you can and look for a physician trained in hypnotherapy, or a hypnotherapist with some sort of medical qualification. Go for self-hypnosis techniques, rather than auto-hypnosis, which relies on an outside stimulus or trigger.

Recently, some of the ideas first proposed by Grantly Dick-Read have provided the inspiration for HypnoBirthing, a technique developed by Marie Mongan, a certified hypnotherapist and hypnoanesthetologist. Mongan's philosophy is summed up by her belief that, "Pizzas are delivered, babies are birthed," and she encourages women to come to terms with their fear, not be overwhelmed by it. HypnoBirthing has a two-pronged approach: it reduces the fear of pain, and then teaches a series of deep relaxation exercises that counteract pain by boosting natural endorphins and suppressing stress hormones and tension.

Have a ball

Formal dress is optional, but you might want to hold a birth ball. These are big rubber physiotherapy balls, a bit like the Spacehopper toys that every child had in the 1970s. In labor, you can sit on them, lean into them, and lean over them for support and counterpressure. You can even take them into the shower. A rolling pin can also be a great massage tool: just get your partner to roll it along your lower back. It also makes a pretty good missile if anyone starts to annoy you. Hollow plastic rolling pins can be filled with hot or cold water, depending on your preference.

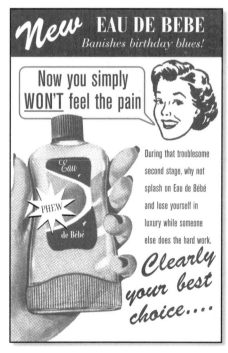

New **EAU DE BEBE**
Banishes birthday blues!

Now you simply WON'T feel the pain

PHEW

During that troublesome second stage, why not splash on Eau de Bébé and lose yourself in luxury while someone else does the hard work.

Clearly your best choice....

Something to sniff at

My idea of aromatherapy is a vapor cloud of Chanel perfume, which might explain why my daughter showed a pronounced and exceedingly precocious preference for it. Some women find the sensory distraction helpful during labor, but don't kid yourself that it will get rid of any pain. The only thing it is guaranteed to get rid of is that underlying smell of stale vomit and disinfectant that clings to many hospitals. This ain't pain relief, but it is a plus point.

If you're convinced of the effectiveness of aromatherapy, then it will probably do some good because the placebo effect comes into play. The best aromatherapy oils are said to be lavender, to restore balance and strengthen contractions; camomile, to calm the mind and body; neroli, to relieve stress; and clary sage, to release muscle tension (but only once you're in labor). These can be added to a birthing pool, or burned in a diffuser. They should never be used neat on the skin because many of them are irritants. They can be diluted with something bland, like jojoba or almond oil.

THE DEAL ON DRUGS AND THEY'RE LEGAL!

Unless there's some sort of emergency, you should call the shots when it comes to the drugs you get in labor. Researchers at the University of Buffalo (presumably men!), described epidurals as "the Cadillac of pain relief." They can be, but a lot depends on who's doing the driving, and how far you've got to travel, so don't rule out other less high-tech options. Why prepare to cross the Rockies when you've only got to get down Rodeo Drive? Anyway, Cadillacs can be murder to park. The same study has also shown that your health insurance, or lack of it, could also affect

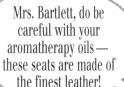

Mrs. Bartlett, do be careful with your aromatherapy oils — these seats are made of the finest leather!

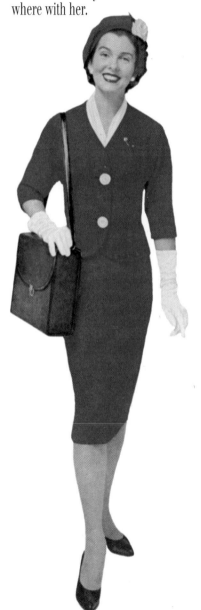

✳ Janet was so thrilled with her mobile epidural that she took it everywhere with her.

what happens. Researchers found that moms with private or HMO coverage were twice as likely to have an epidural for a straightforward vaginal delivery as Medicaid moms. When it comes to C-sections, Medicaid moms are twice as likely to be knocked out with a general anesthetic, rather than being given an epidural so that they can see the baby's arrival. The study revealed ethnic divides, too. Caucasian women are much more likely to get an epidural for either a vaginal or Cesarean delivery than African-Americans. No one's saying this picture applies across the board, but just be aware that it could color your corner of the world.

Epidurals

An epidural block, or lumbar epidural as it's also known, is relatively safe and very effective. Early studies suggested they increased the risk of backache, but this has not been supported by more recent research. A tiny needle or catheter is used to inject local anesthetic into the epidural space above the membrane covering the spinal cord and the bones surrounding it. This numbs the nerves coming from the lower spine that go to the uterus, vagina, and perineum or pelvic floor. Older style epidurals used large doses and heavy-duty motor-blocking, which caused greater numbness. If possible, go for one of the newer "walking" or "mobile" epidurals, which leave you with some movement and a lot more dignity when it comes to peeing. The amount of anesthetic used depends on what stage of labor you're at and your build. As well as anesthetics, it's also possible to administer narcotics through the catheter. This may cause itching—but a lot of moms say it's worth it for the pain relief. You can't have an epidural if you have spinal abnormalities or any sort of bleeding disorder, but it's particularly useful if the baby's in an awkward position or there's more than one in there.

If you're having one, you'll be asked to lie on your side, curled up in a fetal position, or to lean forward over a chair or bed. The skin is cleaned and

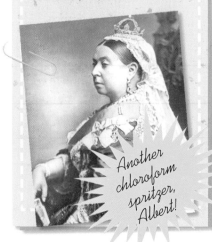

Hurrah for Vicky!

The idea of pain relief during childbirth took a while to catch on. For many years, doctors—all male, of course—opposed the idea. It wasn't widely accepted until Britain's Queen Victoria (1819–1901), the one who wasn't amused—and who would be after nine children?—insisted on pain relief for number seven. It came in the form of chloroform, dripped onto something that looked like a strainer with a hanky in the middle. Once Vicky had given chloroform the thumbs up, this gave the green light to more improvements.

Another chloroform spritzer, Albert!

numbed with local anesthetic before a needle is inserted into the epidural space. At this point it's really important that you stay absolutely still, because if the anesthetist hits the dura (a membrane covering the spinal cord) or one of the tiny veins in the space, there could be complications (in about one percent of cases, epidurals can cause a spinal "headache"—a bad headache that worsens with a change in position). Once the needle is in, you'll be given either a single shot or a dripfeed of anesthetic. You won't feel this at the time, but later on it can hurt like hell.

After a Cesarean, a type of morphine known as duramorph is used through the epidural or spinal to get 24 more hours of pain relief and this makes it easier to get up and breast-feed. One side effect of any epidural is that your blood pressure may drop, so before the epidural an IV line is often put in to keep you hydrated. With the older style epidurals or denser blocks, the urge to push is reduced, so you may be more likely to need forceps or a vacuum delivery, though this is debatable. Madeleine, 24, says, "Next time I'm going to try to do it without the epidural, because I've had a backache ever since. My physician said it's got nothing to do with the epidural, it's just one of those things that happen when you have babies, but I'm not convinced and it definitely slowed up my ability to push."

Blocks

These are local anesthetics that block a particular bunch of nerves. In the past, pudendal blocks were used to knock out the lower section of the vagina, but these are rarely used nowadays. Perineal blocks, which numb the bit between your vagina and butt, are more common, and are often used before an episiotomy or before repairing a tear. Anesthetic is injected directly into the area and will last for around 90 minutes.

The IV league

Analgesics such as Demerol are most often used during the early stages of labor or just after delivery. They're given as an IV drip or as a single shot into a bit of muscle, usually your butt—or a combination of both. They dull the entire nervous system, and muffle sensations so that pain is reduced to a feeling of pressure. Analgesics given as shots take up to 30 minutes to kick in, so don't expect instant pain relief, but with an IV drip the effect is immediate. They can make you feel dizzy or nauseous (which is why they're often given with anti-nausea medication). The biggest drawback is that they cross the placenta, and if they're given too close to the delivery, your baby might arrive drowsy, with breathing difficulties, showing no interest in sucking, and with poor reflexes. This can be fixed with extra oxygen or a shot of another drug, Narcan. Another drawback is that they do not provide great pain relief during active labor.

Wake me up when it's over

General anesthetics should be confined to emergencies, but the Buffalo study (*see page 128*) suggests that there are financial considerations, too. Some women really don't want to know what's going on during delivery at all and are delighted to be put out for the count, but if you'd like to see your baby's arrival, request an epidural if possible. The biggest risk is doing a Janis Joplin and choking on your own vomit, which is why you're asked not to eat or drink too much during labor. You'll be given a shot to knock you out and then a muscle relaxant, which enables the anesthetist to push a tube down your throat to pump in the anesthetic gases. You might feel drowsy and nauseous when you wake up, and have a sore throat.

Nose-breathing for a Drugfree Birth

Doctors prove that women who breathe through their noses throughout birth need no further pain relief. Buy Dr. Dumb's report now.

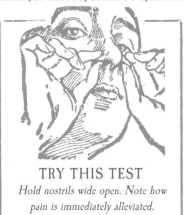

TRY THIS TEST
Hold nostrils wide open. Note how pain is immediately alleviated.

GIVE IT YOUR BREAST SHOT

Breastmilk is free; it never runs out; you don't have to mix it up and sterilize bottles; and there's also evidence to suggest that the babies who drink it are smarter, healthier, and have stronger immune systems. Studies have also shown that as adults, they have lower rates of heart disease, diabetes, and strokes. Moms who breast-feed are less likely to get breast and ovarian cancers. So why on earth is there any debate about the benefits of breast-feeding, and why do so many moms stop so soon?

✳ *This is all for your benefit, Junior, and when you grow up, you're gonna owe me big time!*

Studies have also shown that breast-fed babies are less likely to be fat, and are less prone to allergies, asthma, tummy upsets, colic, glue ear, constipation, the runs, Crohn's disease, and childhood cancers. They are also less likely to succumb to crib death.

Women and their babies started hitting the bottle at around the same time that childbirth became something that happened in hospitals. There was an element of emancipation in bottle-feeding, because moms could leave their babies and do something really shocking, like go out to work. Bottle-feeding also fitted into the new male-oriented view of maternity as a medical condition that had to be managed. It suited hospital routines, which had been set up for the convenience of the doctors and nurses who ran communal nurseries, rather than for the benefit of the babies who were banished to them. Maybe there was even an element of breast envy. As a result, by the 1950s only a few diehards and bohemians were brave enough to buck the trend, and those who did were usually regarded as being a few drops short of a pint. Anyone brave enough to bare their boobies in public faced appalling abuse; many were banished to the bathroom. Even in the 1990s, women in many states were threatened with indecency charges for daring to breast-feed in public. Now, that really is indecent!

In the 1970s, women discovered feminism, burned their bras, and started breast-feeding again. The fact that these latter two activities became popular at around the same time probably explains why

I've never had any problem with breast-feeding in public.

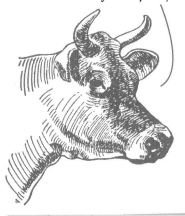

Inverted nipples

If your nipples stick out when it's really cold, or when you're really hot, they're probably not inverted. They should also stick out a bit more as the pregnancy progresses. To find out if you have introverts or extroverts, squeeze the base of the nipple gently with your thumb and forefinger. If it tries to head for cover, you have inverted nipples. There are plastic shields that you can wear during pregnancy to try to tease them out, or you can ask your partner for a little mouth-to-mammary resuscitation.

so many people believe the myth that your boobies have to head south when you breast-feed. Nowadays, two out of three moms at least give it a try, but only one-third are still providing meals on heels at six months. The Government's Healthy People 2010 goal is for 75 percent of moms to start, and at least 50 percent to stick with it for five to six months, so there's still a long way to go.

When it comes to advice, the simple way to sort the milch cows from the silly cows is to ask the woman offering it whether she did actually breast-feed, and, if so, for how long. This includes health professionals, because you'd be amazed how many female obstetricians and pediatricians don't go with the flow. Some of the silliest reasons not to breast-feed tend to come from older women who used bottles. Be warned, this could include your mom. "Oh no, dear, breast milk is too rich," is one such pearl of idiocy. Such advice is usually followed by a long list of foods that you shouldn't eat while breast-feeding, probably including apples, cabbage, cheese, grapes, oranges, strawberries, beans, spicy food, and garlic. Then there are terrifying lists of things like coffee, alcohol, and nicotine that could supposedly Mickey Finn your milk supply and turn your newborn into a chainsmoking lush who likes staying up late. Yes, of course it's best not to smoke while you're breast-feeding, but that doesn't mean that bottle-feeding is better: it isn't.

If you do decide to breast-feed, the first milk you'll make won't actually be milk—it's a yellow liquid called colostrum, which is bursting with proteins, vitamins, and disease-fighting immunoglobulins. You'll start making mature breast milk some time around Day Two or Three. Some people say this milk "comes in," which makes it sound like that purse you ordered is now in stock. In reality it can be a bit uncomfortable around this time because your boobies, brain, and baby are still trying to sort out how much milk to make and when to ship it to the pumping

ESSENTIALS

HIDDEN BENEFITS

Scientists have discovered that breast-fed babies and bottle-fed babies grow very different types of digestive bacteria—and this may explain why breast is best.

Poop analysis shows that breast-fed babies have higher levels of some bugs called bifidobacteria, which are associated with a lower risk of gastric infections and allergy.

Some studies show that these friendly bacteria release natural antibiotics which help fight infection. There's good evidence, too that having a lot of bifidobacteria in their belly means your baby is much less likely to get eczema, asthma, and other allergies.

Bottle-fed babies, however, have fewer bifidobacteria and more clostridia—a not-so-friendly bacteria that is associated with a higher risk of allergy, tummy upsets, and other health problems. Some formula manufacturers are now developing products that both encourage the growth of bacteria already living in the digestive system (prebiotics), and contain live friendly bacteria (probiotics).

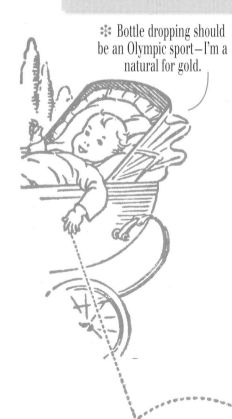

❋ Bottle dropping should be an Olympic sport—I'm a natural for gold.

station. The good news is that you'll have a cleavage to die for and the discomfort doesn't last for long because feeding on demand will quickly sort out any of these supply blips.

There are many reasons why women don't try, or give up. You should definitely use bottles if you're HIV positive, are taking prescription medicines that could hurt your baby, or have a serious drug or drink problem. It may be difficult (but not impossible) to breast-feed if your nipples are inverted, if you have had breast reduction surgery, a difficult labor, or if you have serious depression. Women who know they're going back to work soon after the birth often go straight to bottles. There are some women who find the whole idea so hideous that they can't bring themselves to even contemplate breast-feeding. The one thing none of these women need is a guilt trip. Try breast-feeding if you can: even if you can manage it for a day or two, it will benefit your baby. However, if you can't face it, or if there are reasons why you shouldn't, that's OK, too. Anyone who says otherwise needs a slap around the face with a wet fish, because forcing yourself to do something you hate is much more harmful than formula feeding.

Equipped for the job

STOCK UP NOW

If you are not going to breast-feed, then you'll need a plentiful supply of bottles and teats, and something with which to sterilize them. Steam sterilizers are simple and safe, but you can also boil bottles, or soak them in a sterilizing solution. Bottles and teats come in all shapes and sizes, but we found that widenecked bottles are best, because you can use them for freezing homemade baby food later on. They're also boobie-shaped. Whatever type of bottle or teat you choose, buy enough of them to provide a day's supply and some to spare. There are no hard and fast rules about this. Recommendations for bottle-feeding—2½ fluid ounces per pound of bodyweight (150 ml per kilo)—are only a rough guide, but human milk can vary a great deal according to diet, mom's health, and all sorts of other factors. If your baby's initial weight loss is more than 10 percent, they're probably not getting enough, but if they've regained their birthweight by Day 10 in the world they're getting plenty. Older babies will soon let you know if they're hungry.

For breast-feeding, you'll need a reasonable intake of healthy food and plenty of drinks, but there's no need to be obsessive about it. More importantly, you'll need patience and a degree of perseverance. Junior could be the ultimate sucker, or could get niggly about latching on. It helps to have a comfy chair, pillows for support, and various things within reach to relieve the boredom while Junior is busy sucking away, such as snacks, drinks, the phone, and remote controls for the TV and sound system. Most experts advise breast-feeding for around six weeks before trying to express milk. When the time's right, look for a battery-operated breast pump that's easy to clean and needs just one hand. You can milk yourself manually, or use a hand-operated pump, but in our book there's no point going economy if you plan to be a frequent flyer.

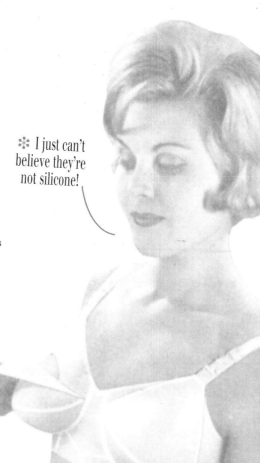

✳ I just can't believe they're not silicone!

BUMPS DON'T MAKE FRUMPS

Why is it that so many maternity clothes make you look like Doris Day on a bad day? She was hardly a role model for maternity: the closest the woman ever got to a sex scene was taking one foot off the floor as she got into bed with Rock Hudson (and he didn't get his rocks off with us girls anyway). Pregnancy changes your life dramatically, but why should it change your wardrobe beyond recognition? "Bump" may rhyme with "frump," but any resemblance should stop right there.

We're not saying that everyone can dress like a supermodel. For starters, supermodels can get paid in kind, so they can barter a few sashays down the runway for cleverly cut frocks that have more shock appeal than schlock repel. However, even if you don't have friends in haute places, there's no excuse for looking like an overstuffed chintz sofa with a Peter Pan collar. You've got to make a few concessions to comfort, like sensible shoes and bigger bras, but there's no reason to change your personal style. There's no denying you've got it, so you might as well flaunt it.

At first, you'll be able to get away with undoing the top button on your jeans and covering the gap with a baggy shirt, or wearing hipster styles that sit neatly under a bump. Some cuts, like empire line, baby doll, and bias cut, make the most of your boobies and still have plenty of room for bumpsie. Sexy can be a hard one to pull off: Liz Hurley tried hard (too hard, some would say) with black stretch lace minis, but there's a fine line between looking terrific and looking like trailer trash. For terrific, see Demi Moore, Sarah Jessica Parker, and Sadie Frost (aka Mrs. Jude Law).

Underpinning is all important. Buy underpants with cotton in the crotch, and head straight for a specialist bra fitter before your cups start running over. Avoid underwiring, as it can cause all sorts of odd bumps and lumps as your boobies grow. Look for styles that offer easy access—like low-cut balconette bras—so that you can use them when breast-

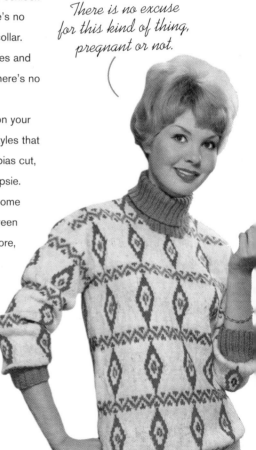

There is no excuse for this kind of thing, pregnant or not.

feeding. The same goes for maternity clothes. You might have a big belly and ass for longer than you'd like, so look for styles that button down the front and leave you room to move.

There's no crime in accessories

Specialist maternity shops are great for special occasions, and suits that show you still mean business, but they can make a big hole in your nesting egg. Those cushions that are meant to indicate how your silhouette will change during your pregnancy are also a complete waste of time, as women can carry so differently. A bulge with more front than Bloomingdales will look completely different than one with a Texan spread. If you're determined to splash out, do it on accessories like designer scarves. They'll cheer up cheap outfits, and you'll still enjoy wearing them when Junior's in school.

Don't be afraid to accept hand-me-downs: if nothing else, they'll relieve the boredom of a limited wardrobe. Make a beeline for chain stores that stock large sizes, and raid your partner's wardrobe for large shirts and waistcoats. If it fits, wear it! Why not head for Bollywood and treat yourself to a salwar kameez or sari? They're glam, gorgeous to wear, and can always be turned into cushion covers or drapes afterward. Scour the classified ads or the Internet for pre-loved maternity clothes, and keep an eye out for garage sales. For the best buys, hunt in neighborhoods with nice family homes and two cars in each driveway. Mail order can be hit and miss: check the fabrics carefully, because a lot of these clothes are made from cheap manmade fibers that are hot to wear and hang like a dish cloth after one or two washes. Buy just one or two items until you're sure that the quality is up to scratch. Give yourself a gold star for buying anything that can be thrown in the washing machine and doesn't need ironing.

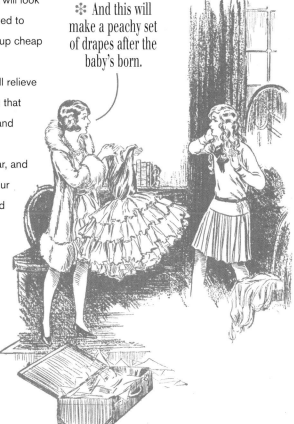

✳ And this will make a peachy set of drapes after the baby's born.

BUY, BUY, BABY

Think sensible when buying for baby. If you've got a bald baby girl, please, please don't buy one of those elasticated headbands saying "I'm a girl!" Everyone who matters knows that already, babies hate wearing them, and they've got all the appeal of an anchovy beached on a hard-cooked egg. Buy very few baby clothes before the birth and bypass the sizes for newborns: most babies grow out of them in a week or two, and some outgrow them before they're even born.

OK Mom, some people think it's unlucky to buy baby clothes before the baby is born, but I am four months old now and getting cold!

Go for a "capsule" wardrobe, so beloved of the stylists: six shirts, six all-in-ones with press-studs that go from the neck right down to both feet, a hat, a couple of pairs of scratch mittens (babies often arrive with talons worthy of a nail parlor, but without the hand control to stop them scratching themselves), and a couple of pairs of booties. You can prolong the life of all-in-ones by cutting out the toes once they become tight. If you live in a Californian climate, you can cut back on the all-in-ones and won't need the socks. If you're in the middle of a Midwest winter, you'll need to add a really good thermal suit to go over everything else, and a couple of jackets.

Babies hate changing their underwear even more than teenage boys do, so always buy garments with wide necks and easy diaper access. Pants that have to come off completely for changes cause more trouble than a chocolate cake at a Weight Watchers meeting. Look for natural fibers, and garments that will stand a hot wash and tumbledrying.

Deals on wheels

Don't be frightened by the mindboggling array of wheels on offer in the nursery department. Apply a few commonsense guidelines and ask the experts—moms with young children—for the real lowdown. Factors that should guide your choice include: the cost; the local terrain; the prevailing weather conditions; how much parking space you have; how many stairs there are to your front door; the height of the handles (you should never have to bend); the size of the wheels and whether they're fixed or not; how much it weighs; and how easy it is to fold up. Factors that shouldn't guide your choice include matching diaper bags, pushy sales assistants, and paparazzi shots of Hollywood moms.

High rollers and rock 'n' rollers

There are two basic designs: baby carriages and strollers. Baby carriages are huge, tend to contain Ivy League offspring, and are often pushed by a nanny in full uniform. Strollers are scaled down versions that are much more suited to the gal about town. Some strollers double as car seats and carriers, and the three-wheeler off-road versions are style statements in some neighborhoods. However, if they never go off-road and you don't have the sporty figure to match, it's a statement that could scream "fashion victim!" Older babies can use lightweight strollers, so you'll probably want to buy one of these later, but they're not suitable for newborns. New babies need to lie down, and it's better if they can face you while doing so (and you will know when it's safe to stop singing "Old MacDonald Had a Farm"). As they get older, and have stronger neck muscles, they like to sit up and watch the world go by: who wouldn't? Strollers that catered for both possibilities were popular with us and our kids. The bigger the wheel, the smoother the ride (and the bigger the turning circle). Big wheels are best for rocky roads, while smaller swivel wheels (sometimes with locking mechanisms) are easier for city living, shopping malls, and smooth suburban sidewalks. If you have to negotiate a flight of stairs to get into your house, go for something with a detachable carry crib. This gives you a fighting chance of getting the baby inside without waking him or her up, which could save your sanity. The weights that are given on the

NO FRILLS

Frills and fancy ties are fine if you like that sort of thing, but long ribbon ties can easily get caught up around your baby's neck and buttons that aren't firmly secured are a sure-fire choking hazard. Give all trimmings and buttons a firm tug to make sure they're firmly sewn on. A tip from an old hand: babies hate getting changed, so keep it simple.

✱ The Kleptocarriage offers plenty of storage space for those impulse acquisitions.

specifications are meaningless. To get a realistic idea of the weight you'll be carrying, add two bags of groceries, one screaming baby, and a diaper bag. Remember that you'll be lifting most of this with one hand while you hold the baby in the other.

Basket cases

A baby basket—or Moses basket—provides a convenient first bed. You can carry it from room to room, and they usually come with collapsible frames that bring them up to bedside level, preventing back injuries during night feedings. Make sure the mattress fits snugly, and use an elasticated liner to protect your baby's head from raffia scratches. If your baby likes to wriggle and squirm up the basket, tuck a blanket under the liner for extra padding (but make sure it can't slip and present a smothering hazard).

Cribs always seem to come in flatpack form with instructions that would make more sense if they'd been translated from the original pygmy by a Japanese-Portuguese dyslexic. Don't wait until your baby's home before you tackle it. Features to look for include: two legs with rollers (two legs mean it's is easier for you to move it, while four legs mean it's easier for Junior to move); an adjustable base (to avoid lifting when baby is little, and lock him or her in later on); and sides that can be lowered and eventually removed. Don't use padded crib bumpers that tie onto the slats, because these can be dangerous.

Is it me, Norma, or do nannies seem to get smaller every day?

Essential extras

DIAPER DEBATES

For some moms, the convenience of disposable diapers outweighs all other considerations. However, "disposable" diapers aren't actually disposable. In ideal conditions they rot away within 50 years, but in some cases they take between 200 and 500 years to decompose. This means that every disposable diaper that has ever been used is still out there, and every day we add a few million more to the poop pile. Ask your mom about cloth diapers and she'll probably need to lie down with a stiff drink, a camomile tea, or a Prozac. In her day it was tough, but nowadays diaper systems make it a lot easier. Most involve biodegradable liners that package up the poop, the diaper, and plastic pants with Velcro fastenings. There's no need for soaking, and modern washing machines blitz most bugs at 140°F (60°C). Diaper services collect the dirties and drop off fresh supplies. Diaper systems are cheaper (and become even more cost effective with siblings), and you can claim vast numbers of ecology plus points if you use them.

Plastic, padded change mats are a must. If you live in a house with more than one floor, have a mat, wipes, and clean diapers on every level. You'll need cotton sheets and blankets for the basket, crib, or stroller; they're easy to wash and less scratchy than wool. You can buy zip-up sleeping bags for use in strollers during really cold weather. Get half a dozen cheesecloth squares for wiping spills, covering up while breast-feeding, and putting over your shoulder to collect baby spitup. Try to get a diaper bag with an outer section that comes off and doubles as a portable changing mat. This is much better than bags that undo and scatter butt cream, wipes, teething gel, and those contraceptives you bought just in case. Plastic baby baths that fit over a standard bath will help to prevent backache.

You'll need a good car seat or baby pod. Don't accept anything secondhand unless you're positive it hasn't been in an accident. Some car seats double as portable seats (which should never be put on tables or anything high), but if you've got one of these, make sure you've had a few stabs at fitting it into the car before the big day when baby comes home. Two hours in the car park is no one's idea of a homecoming. Be careful when buying baby slings and carriers that strap to your body. Some of them offer less support than a lazy shrink, and you'll end up holding the baby anyway. Look for something that distributes the baby's weight evenly, and has plenty of padding on the straps. For the best advice, ask a physical therapist.

Travel cribs are handy when visiting baby's adoring fans, and they double as play pens. You can also get portable high chairs that screw onto the table, or are secured by the baby's own weight. Baby walkers might look like fun, but they're really bad news. They delay walking, provide babies with better access to all sorts of dangerous stuff, and provide overtime for hospital emergency rooms.

VACATION OPTIONS

Take a decent break during your pregnancy. It might seem like an indulgence now, but when you're surrounded by dirty diapers, you'll be glad that you have a few pleasure points in the bank. So long as there are no added risk factors such as bleeding, really bad anemia, high blood pressure, or a previous miscarriage, there's no good reason to stay at home. Ignore the killjoys who think you shouldn't go any further than the corner store. These are the same people who call pregnancy "confinement."

✳ Enjoying yourself when pregnant is not what we doctors would advise!

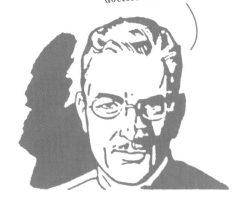

INSURANCE

If you're going abroad, take out a top-of-the-line travel insurance policy, read the fine print, and make sure it covers cancellation costs if a complication crops up before you leave. It's bad enough losing out on the vacation, without losing the cash as well.

Let commonsense be your tour guide. Backpacking or whitewater rafting are great when you're big on adventure and full of energy. However, now you are big of belly and full of fetus, and there's a lot to be said for modern bathrooms, air-conditioning, and basic hygiene standards. Choose a destination that has adequate obstetric care and an excellent hospital. Avoid really hot places now that your body temperature is a bit higher than usual anyway, and altitudes above 6,500 feet (2,000 m) unless you're used to such conditions. Don't fly on unpressurized aircraft. Big planes are OK, but the little aircraft that hop around the Caribbean and the Mediterranean aren't.

Ask your doctor or a government agency for safe travel advice. Vaccinations will rule out a lot of destinations: most shots should be avoided in the first 12 weeks, and by the time you've had the full course, airlines may be getting nervous about letting you onboard. Most airlines won't let you fly in the last two months. If you look big, they could refuse to take you on board earlier, so take a letter from your doctor confirming your dates. It's also useful to carry a copy of your medical notes and a medical phrasebook: you never know when you'll need to say "hemorrhoids" or "placenta." Ask your doctor or travel agent to recommend a local doctor. Some health insurers provide lists. Take a medical kit, including antacids, painkillers, diarrhea medicine, and insect repellents that are safe to use during pregnancy. Add some packages of rehydrating salts, or make your own by adding a pinch of salt and a teaspoon of sugar to 2 pints (950 ml) of cooled, boiled water.

Water works

When local water supplies are suspect, drink only bottled water, and always check that the seal is intact. If you're suffering from heartburn or indigestion, look for mineral water with a high level of bicarbonate. Use bottled water to brush your teeth and to wash any fruit that can't be peeled. Avoid salads, ice in drinks, and buffets with stale food. Don't risk foods from street vendors, particularly ice cream. Avoid undercooked meat and burgers at all times.

Tips for planes, trains, and automobiles

Long-haul flights can be a pain in the butt, among other places. Swollen ankles and cramps tend to get worse when you have minimal oxygen and legroom. This combination also increases the chance of deep vein thrombosis (a blood clot that starts as a dull ache and can end in a fatal stroke). Drink plenty of fluids (not alcohol), take regular walks, and wear tight socks or elasticated compression stockings. Try to get an aisle seat near the toilets, preferably at the front of the aircraft because it's less of a hassle getting on and off and the air quality's better. If you get dizzy, ask a steward for extra oxygen. Find out how busy the flight is when checking in, and ask if there's a chance of leaving the seat next to you empty. If you say you're scared of throwing up over another passenger, you'll go to the top of the line.

Trains can be civilized, if a little slow. There is plenty of legroom, space to stroll around, and easy access to the john. There might even be an onboard buffet, although you're unlikely to discover anything particularly nutritious in it.

When you're traveling by car, take plenty of pit stops. Use a pillow to support the small of your back, and carry a coolbag with drinks and snacks. Some women like to sit on a towel in case their waters break. When wearing a seatbelt, be careful to tuck the lap section under your bump, and the diagonal between your boobies and your belly.

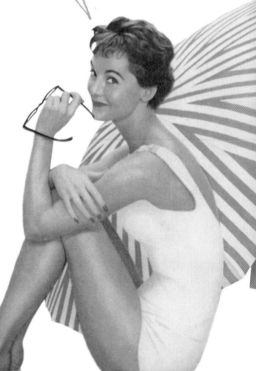

Pay no attention to old Dr. Misery, he's just jealous that I'm in Paradise and he's in Poughkeepsie.

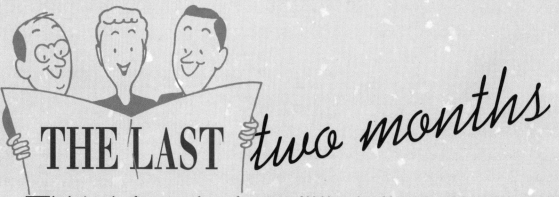

THE LAST *two months*

The last weeks of pregnancy have a funny way of kicking a lot of fears about labor into touch. When you're the size of Montana, bits of your body stop working properly, and you're peeing so often you should buy shares in the local water company, there are some days that labor pains don't look so bad. Then you catch sight of your stomach and say, "How on earth am I going to get this out?"

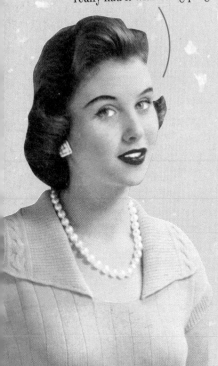

✳ You may not think it to look at me, but I have really, really, really, really had it with being pregnant.

IIt's always on one of these days that you run into an old school friend with five kids and endless childbirth stories, all of which seem to involve marathon labours, more instruments than the London Philharmonic and blood loss on the scale of the Texas Chainsaw Massacre. Sometimes it's hard to know whether that feeling gripping your innards is sheer terror or just another Braxton Hicks.

One minute you won't be able to stand the thought of another day of pregnancy, and the next you won't be able to stand the thought of the labour actually starting. Crossing your legs isn't an option. You might feel anxious, bored, calm, desperate, edgy, fed up, grumpy, hysterical, impatient, jittery, knowing, lethargic, moody, nervous, overwrought, paranoid, queasy, restive, scared, tense, uptight, vulnerable, worried, yearning, X-rated and zonked — all on the same day.

There are 101 reasons why the last weeks of pregnancy can be a drag — more details about those soon. You will have forgotten how to go half an hour without wondering where the toilet is, being able to sit with your knees together, what it feels like to get a good night's sleep, what your feet look like and how to walk without looking like a demented penguin.

The only thing you won't forget is how many days there are until your due date — you'll be counting them off like a kid at Christmas time.

The name game is one way to kill some time and develop all sorts of homicidal thoughts about partners, mums, mums-in-law and other family members, who might have their own firm views on names. If you choose a family name, you risk offending one side of the family. If you choose a name that's really popular, you'll keep running into kids with the same name. If you go for something out of the ordinary, you might be providing ammunition for playground bullies. Blame it on the hormones or exhaustion, but after a while the strangest names start to sound half sensible: we know of one couple who convinced themselves that Shirt would make a great name for a boy. Mercifully, they had a girl! If you name a boy Sue, he'll probably do just that, citing mental cruelty and child abuse. For inspiration, and a few laughs, borrow or buy one of those books of names and their meanings, look at film credits, and flick through favorite novels. If you're going to get all literary, make sure you've got the spelling right: Porsche is the car manufacturer, Portia is the babe in *The Merchant of Venice*. Other pitfalls include abbreviations and acronyms: Tommy Indiana Turner might have a nice ring to it, but it will get on your son's TITs, while Barbara Ursula Maddox could have a really BUM time at school.

When you're heavy with child, you need a little light relief. Pull out your birth plan: it could provide some belly laughs. The priorities you had in the early months — like checking the feng shui of the labour room, having your lip gloss within reach at all times and asking for the anaesthetist who looks like Mel Gibson — might not seem quite so important now. Your options may also have changed as a result of complications such as stalled weight gain (the baby's, not yours), hypertension or gestational diabetes.

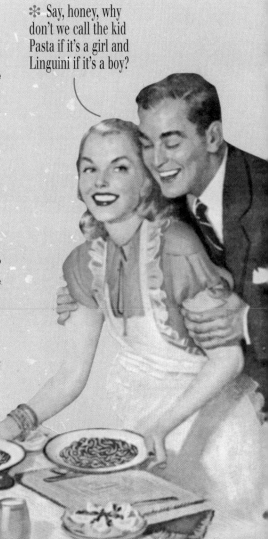

✷ Say, honey, why don't we call the kid Pasta if it's a girl and Linguini if it's a boy?

SO YOU'RE SICK OF BEING PREGNANT

As well as being apprehensive about labor, you'll find that the last weeks of pregnancy can throw up a whole host of unwanted extras to drive you crazy. If the constipation, heartburn, varicose veins, and Braxton Hicks don't get you, then the nosebleeds, hemorrhoids, breathlessness, indigestion, and backache probably will. Here's a rundown of all the crappy things that you might be going through, and, more importantly, a few tips that might help to keep you sane.

Aches AND STRAINS

Pregnancy can be a pain in the neck, back, and butt. In fact, it can be a pain just about anywhere. Relaxin—the cool dude hormone (*see page 30 and page 102*)—makes everything hang loose, so your ligaments provide as much support as an old bra that's been through the wash once too often. Whenever you take exercise—assuming that you can face it by this stage—be careful to warm up and cool down properly to avoid strains.

Most women get a backache to some degree. Swimming strengthens and supports your back muscles, and provides a rare opportunity to feel light and fantastic: even hippos look graceful in the water. On dry land, watch your posture, and send the stilettos or kitten heels into hibernation. If there's something heavy to lift, bend from your knees (or, even better, get someone else to do it—consider it one of the perks of the condition). Act like one of the guys: put your feet up at every opportunity. Gentle massage and heat pads might help, and see a physical therapist if it gets really bad. Remember that babies become even more backbreaking once they're on the outside.

Abdominal pains

These can be caused by ligaments and muscles being stretched further than Bill Clinton's credibility when he denied sexual relations with Monica Lewinsky. You might experience aches and cramps, or

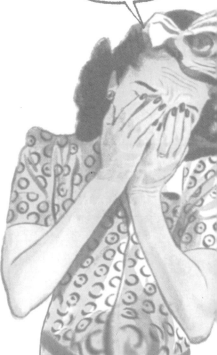

One more patronizing pregnancy book and I swear I will break my own water!

short stabs of pain, particularly when you're getting out of a chair, bed, or car, or having a good cough or laugh. There's no need to worry, so long as they don't become a frequent fixture and there are no other warning signs, like dizziness, fever, chills, vaginal discharge, or bleeding.

Braxton Hicks

These are the practice contractions that can start as early as 20 weeks, particularly if you've been around the baby block before. One minute you'll be gazing longingly at the Ben and Jerry's cabinet, and the next you'll feel— and sometimes even see—your belly tighten up quicker than a miser's money belt when the restaurant check arrives. This is caused by your uterus flexing its muscles and limbering up for the big day. Braxton Hicks contractions don't last long—two minutes at most, and usually about 30 seconds—and most of the time they don't hurt. As D-Day approaches, they will become more frequent and intense, and may start to hurt like hell. It's not labor, but sometimes it's really hard to tell. Always mention them to your healthcare provider. Get advice right away if you get more than four an hour, or if you also have back pain, or if your briefs are wet from any abnormal fluid or discharge.

Constipation

Some women spend more time and energy pushing because of constipation than they ever do in labor, but this is misguided: the act of pushing will actually tighten up your butt and make it even more difficult to dump a load. To combat constipation, make sure that you eat more fiber and drink more fluids. Instead of straining, try to relax your ring and visualize it gently opening out. Squatting on the seat instead of sitting can also get things moving, but watch your balance. At home, use a steady chair for support; when you're out, use handicap johns with grab rails.

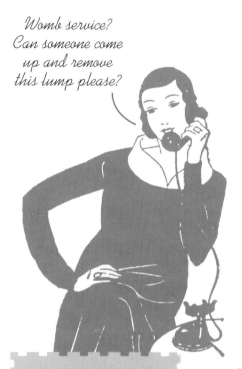

Womb service? Can someone come up and remove this lump please?

BREATHLESSNESS

Breathlessness that would make Marilyn Monroe blush is caused by extra blood, extra weight, and the extra work your heart is doing to keep everything circulating. Your lungs work differently during pregnancy, and are able to take in more oxygen than normal, so there's no need to worry unless you go blue at the lips and fingertips.

Carpal tunnel syndrome

This is another name for pins and needles in your hands, particularly in the morning. It's caused by fluid retention, which squishes the nerves. Some doctors recommend sleeping with your hands propped up on a pillow, but they don't say how you're meant to keep them there in your sleep. If it's bad, try sleeping with strap-on wrist splints. Alternatively, put your hands above your head for a few minutes when you first wake up, allowing some of the extra fluid to drain away.

> Euw! Believe me, readers, you do not want to see what has happened to my ankles!

Cramps

If cramps are your style, drink extra fluids and try leg circling exercises in a warm bath before bedtime (this gives sluggish circulation a kick in the butt). For a do-it-yourself foot massage, put a bottle or tennis ball on the floor and roll it back and forth with the sole of your foot. Eat bananas: they're packed with potassium, which helps to prevent cramps. Extra vitamin B or calcium might also help.

WATER WORKS

Dropsy

Your mom might call this "fluid retention." (It's also a good reason not to pick up fragile ornaments, anything by Lalique, and your best friend's new crystal.) It might sound a bit strange, but the best thing for fluid retention is more fluid, preferably something healthy such as water, juice, or milk. For more tips, see edema, opposite.

Dropping your bundle

If you have a flabby pelvic floor or have had children before, you might feel as if your baby's about to slip out. This is rarely a problem the first time around, but let it be a warning about the importance of doing your Kegel exercises to keep your pelvic floor in good shape (see pages 98–101).

Fainting

Fainting or feeling dizzy when lying on your back affects one in ten heavily pregnant women, and it's all to do with the inferior vena cava. This is a big artery running down your back, and it gets squashed by all that extra uterus, baby, placenta, and amniotic fluid. As soon you turn onto your side, the faintness will pass. Early in pregnancy, the extra blood and stretchy veins can also cause faintness. Avoid standing for long periods, and try to sit down before you fall down.

✳ Rhoda's fainting fits always happened when Errol was around.

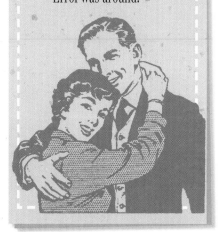

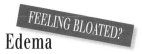

Edema

This is the term for all that extra fluid that hangs around your ankles and hands, making rings and shoes uncomfortable. Drink more, not less, liquid to flush it out, and take off any rings or bangles that are getting too tight for comfort. If you're a hopeless romantic or a rockaholic, consider this: it's better than having your jewelry cut off because your fingers are turning blue and threatening to drop off. Don't take diuretics, not even the herbal ones like dandelion root tea: they affect blood flow across the placenta, and could mask pre-eclampsia. Always mention edema to your doctor or nurse-midwife.

Exhaustion

This makes a comeback in the final weeks, but at least your size is now in proportion to your sloth. Don't fight it, get as much rest as you can.

Ears

Your ears might pick up funny whooshy noises, or amplify your heartbeat. It's OK, you're not receiving communications from extraterrestrials. It's probably caused by the extra blood volume and stretchy veins, and it goes away once the baby's born.

Gums

Your gums might bleed so much that they should carry a donor card. You will need a softer toothbrush, dental floss, and a dental descale. Extra blood and pregnancy hormones will make gums more spongy and prone to bleeding, but the underlying problem is usually a buildup of plaque. Don't delay going to the dentist: researchers at Case Western Reserve University in Cleveland found that there is some truth in the old wives' tale that you'll lose a tooth for every pregnancy, but infection (rather than calcium loss) appears to be the problem. Dental infections can spread, and might harm your baby or your heart, so ask your doctor if you need antibiotics before any work is done. *See also* "Pregnancy tumors" *on page 153.*

"Pregnancy tumors" *on page 153.*

Headaches

You obviously didn't have a headache roughly nine months ago, but you might get them throughout the pregnancy. An occasional acetaminophen is OK, but aspirin is a no-no. Late in pregnancy, headaches could be a sign of pre-eclampsia, and should always be checked out. Drug-free approaches that are worth a try include cold compresses, massaging your temples with a little lavender oil diluted with a neutral carrier oil such as almond oil, and visualization—which is just a fancy way of saying you psyche it away. It's a neat trick that can work for lots of minor aches and pains. Just take a few minutes out to relax, and give your pain or problem a visual image—creases that need ironing out, brambles that have to be dug out of the backyard, or grit that should be swept away, whatever—and then draw a mental picture of it happening. OK, we know that sounds ludicrously simple, but if you can maintain your focus and concentration it really does work.

Heartburn and indigestion

Backdrafts that would floor a fireman are caused by relaxin, which softens up the valve that should stop stomach acid gurgling back up your windpipe. The fact that Junior is pushing up into your stomach only adds to the pressure and the indigestion. Drinking milk might help, and most antacids are OK, but watch the sugar content, particularly if you have any form of diabetes. At bedtime, prop yourself up with an extra pillow. Heartburn usually eases off when Junior becomes "engaged" and slips down into the launch position.

HICCUPS

Some babies get hiccups so often that you'll start wondering what's in the amniotic fluid. These can be disconcerting. Attacks can last for up to half an hour, but they'll bug you more than your baby.

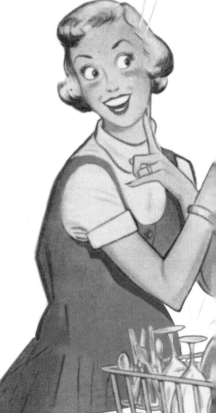

Hemorrhoids

These are a real pain in the butt. Suddenly all those television commercials that show people wincing and looking sheepish won't seem so hilarious any more. Try to eat more fiber and drink plenty of fluids to avoid constipation, and try not to push when you poop (*see also* Constipation, *page 147*). Drugstore remedies will relieve the itch. If they're painful, try sitting on a bag of frozen peas. If you're bleeding heavily or suffering unbearable pain, contact you doctor.

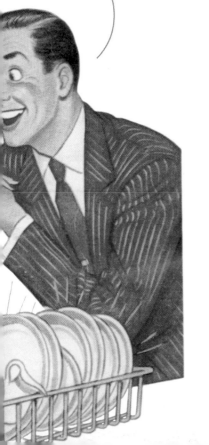

✳ You see, sweetpea. Didn't I tell you that doing the whole block's dishes would cure your itchy little digits?

Irritability

Don't be fooled by the gooey pictures of women looking serenely beautiful in pregnancy magazines: there'll be times when you look—and feel—like Alice Cooper on a bad day. It's OK, it's allowed! Forget the soft-focus garbage: there are plenty of good reasons for feeling ghastly. Count to ten or take six deep breaths before biting off your partner's head—and steer clear of live chickens.

Itching

Itchy hands and feet may be signs of intrahepatic cholestasis of pregnancy, which means that your liver's not working properly. The itching can be really bad: your hands might feel as if they're on fire, and it's not uncommon for women to scratch until they bleed. It causes jaundice in moms, and increases the risk of stillbirth. If you're worried, ask your doctor or nurse-midwife to arrange a blood test: treatment is available. Most itching is much more mundane. Itchy bellies are usually caused by the skin being stretched tight. Thrush and diabetes cause vaginal itches, as can underwear that's not made from cotton, and scented soaps. An itchy, or highly sensitive, clitoris is also quite common, and is caused by all the extra blood glugging around your body.

Leukorrhoea

LEUKO WHAT?

This is the medical term for that gush of thin white non-smelling discharge, which occurs during pregnancy and makes you feel as if you've peed your pants. It may also be a sign of your waters breaking, so contact your carer if you're concerned. Just change your briefs more frequently, and avoid using scented soaps or any sort of vaginal spray or deodorant because this will only aggravate the problem.

Moods

In the last few weeks, your moods will swing more than a party at the Playboy mansion. Don't beat yourself up if you get the blues: you don't have to be blissful and Madonna-like (the first one, not the Material Girl). If you talk to other moms-to-be, you'll probably find that you're not alone and things aren't so bad. There's always bound to be someone else whose hypertension is worse, or whose bathroom is even more of a building site.

Migraines

These are often worst in the first trimester and then tend to improve, but if they were linked to your periods before pregnancy, you're much less likely to get a break. If you are experiencing migraines talk to your doctor. Some migraine medications are not advisable, but products containing acetaminophen are OK, and cold compresses help if you apply them as soon as the attack starts.

Noses

These get clogged up with extra mucus, and have a nasty habit of bleeding because of the extra blood and pregnancy hormones. Try pinching the nose at the bridge, or put something really cold over it to stem the flow. Saline drops may also help.

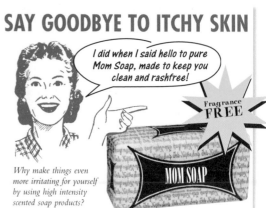

SAY GOODBYE TO ITCHY SKIN

I did when I said hello to pure Mom Soap, made to keep you clean and rashfree!

Fragrance **FREE**

MOM SOAP

Why make things even more irritating for yourself by using high intensity scented soap products?

KICKING

K is for kicking and kidneys, a combination that babies love and you'll soon learn to hate. Babies have a habit of kicking you when you're down, or in any other position they don't happen to like. Eventually they run out of room in which to really let loose, but some women find this even more disconcerting, and worry that something's gone wrong. *See kick charts, page 89.*

Overheating and overeating

Overheating during the last two months is unavoidable because of the extra blood and the extra load on board. Wear loose clothes in natural fibers, and take plenty of cool showers and baths. Overeating is almost impossible, because your stomach is being scrunched up by the extra uterus and baby, particularly if you're carrying high.

Pregnancy tumors

These aren't tumors at all, but yet another example of how dumb doctors can be when it comes to names. They are little nodules that grow out of gums, and occasionally on other bits of your body. They also go by the name of pyogenic granulomas, which doesn't have much of a ring to it either. They bleed easily, but look a lot worse than they really are. They usually go away after the birth, but you can have them cut off if they're a real nuisance.

Perspiration

The amount of perspiration increases, and you might feel as if your entire body has sprung a leak. This can cause heat rash, but it won't smell as much as you'd think, because you'll be sweating all over, not just at the stinky bits under the arms and boobies and around the crotch.

Queasiness

Q is for queasiness, which usually tails off by the end of the first trimester. However, some unlucky women suffer from beginning to end. The sight of Hollywood moms squeezing into size 6 jeans a week after they give birth is also enough to trigger a relapse. For tips on coping with morning sickness, *see pages 36–39.*

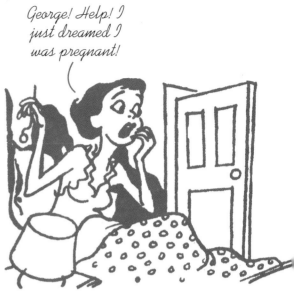

George! Help! I just dreamed I was pregnant!

NIGHTMARES

Horror films will be nothing compared to some of the stuff your brain dreams up in the last weeks of pregnancy, like giving birth to a monster, or putting the pot roast to bed and the baby on to boil. Freudians have their own interpretations: for instance, dreams of being trapped or drowning are supposed to signify worries about the loss of freedom. Some women find this approach helpful, and like to jot down and analyze the bits they can remember. Others prefer to let their sleeping neuroses lie.

NO ROOM AT THE INN

Rib stitch

Rib stitches and pains are caused by the baby pushing up into your chest and stretching your rib cage. As space starts to run out, babies often shove their feet right into the middle of the ribs, where the stomach used to be. Sometimes, changing position or wriggling around will persuade Junior to move, but basically there's not a lot you can do. It will ease off toward the end, when your baby's head slips into your pelvis and becomes "engaged"—always a cause for celebration.

✳ Be careful in there, sugar—they say that rib stitch can be really uncomfortable.

✳ Nonsense darling, I've been wearing this for weeks and I can feel a thing.

Red markings

Red markings that run along veins and hurt when you touch them could be blood clots, aka thrombosis. Shallow surface clots occur in around one in 50 pregnancies, and although they're not as dangerous as deep vein thrombosis, they do need to be dispersed. Treatments include rest, putting your feet up, ointments, and wearing compression stockings.

Stretch marks

These red marks burst forth on bellies, butts, and thighs. Save yourself a fortune, and forget all those fancy creams with French names and scientific ingredients. The only things that set them apart from a good budget moisturizer are the price and the packaging. Creams moisturize the skin's surface, but can't get to the deeper layers where the real damage is being done. The only thing that will prevent stretch marks is having the right genes, and you can't buy these at the cosmetic counter.

Sleep

Sleep is harder to get than a cab after the office Christmas party. If cramps and indigestion don't keep you awake, the weight of bumpsie and having to get up for a pee probably will. Put pillows under your belly, between your knees, under your feet, and anywhere else that helps. Try a lettuce sandwich washed down with warm milk to obtain some natural soporifics.

Tags

These are little bits of extra skin that pop out in high-friction areas like the underarms, around bras (particularly if you ignored advice about avoiding underwire styles), and at the top of the legs. They'll probably go away, but if they're in an uncomfortable spot you can have them snipped off.

Urination

You've been posted with the Pee Corps. The urination rate slows down for a while during the midterm, but towards the end there's so little room to move down there that your bladder's capacity is severely curtailed. You'll have to get up at least once in the night for a pee.

Varicose veins

Varicose veins can make your legs look like a road map of Manhattan. The fine little ones usually disappear of their own accord, but the bigger blue ones that bulge out and sprout nobbly little eruptions can be quite painful. Avoid standing for long periods, and wear support stockings—they can be custom-made if necessary and come in a variety of colors (it's best to put them on after lying down so the blood will not pool in the legs). A less appealing, but nonetheless comforting, look is to wrap your legs in a damp towel and put your feet up as soon as you get home. This also gets you out of cooking dinner.

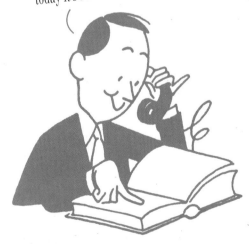

❄ We had Chinese yesterday and Indian the day before, so today it's PIZZA!

CODE RED CONDITIONS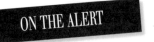

I f you think that the minor league of pregnancy problems can pitch a few curve balls, keep your fingers crossed that you don't make it into the major league, which sends down bean balls like bleeding, high blood pressure, and leaks of amniotic fluid. These can all be as scary as they sound, but the odds of serious pregnancy problems happening are somewhere between a blind date with Tom Cruise and being given a Versace original at your baby shower, and prompt medical care can often defuse the crisis.

If you have any of the following symptoms, see a doctor or nurse-midwife immediately. They'd much rather deal with nervous paranoia than a major medical emergency. Any bright red blood requires immediate action: it may mean something is wrong with the placenta. A very small amount of blood in a jellylike plug could be the "show" at the start of labor. Swelling, really bad headaches, seeing spots or lights before your eyes, twitching, pain at the top of your belly, feeling sleepy, and reflex reactions that have gone into overdrive are signs of pre-eclampsia (see pages 76–77).

Heavy, painful, or very swollen calves could be signs of deep vein thrombosis (DVT), a type of blood clot. The blockage is rarely visible, but smaller veins near the surface may look fatter and darker than usual, because your blood supply is using them as detours to avoid the jam. It also hurts more when you point your toes up toward your chin. DVTs are most common just before and after the birth, because one of our body's survival tricks is to make blood a bit thicker so that we don't bleed buckets during delivery.

High fever may mean an infection, which could spread to the baby and is sometimes, but not always, associated with an infection of the amniotic fluid. If this has happened, treatment will depend on where you're at in the pregnancy calendar, but beware: infection can make your baby sick and trigger premature labor, so any warning signs should always be checked out. Abdominal tenderness can also be a sign of infection in the amniotic fluid, or that the placenta is breaking away from the uterus ahead of schedule.

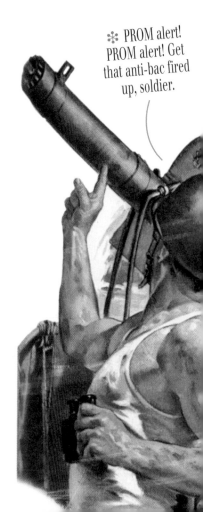

✳ PROM alert! PROM alert! Get that anti-bac fired up, soldier.

HOLD FIRE

Reading through lists of all the stuff that can go wrong can blow minor niggles into full-scale emergencies—in your mind, that is. On the frontline, the first rule is DON'T PANIC, and it's no different in the frontline of pregnancy. If any of this is ringing alarm bells, take six deep breaths, think skeptical, and think again. If you're still worried after all that, call for help.

✳ Sir, yes sir! But we're going to need a lot more broad spectrum ammo.

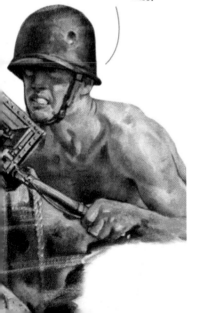

Waters-gate and the lowdown on leaks

The bubble of fluid that surrounds your baby is not meant to burst until labor starts, but some women spring a leak much earlier, and start to drip or gush more than a lady who lunches. It's known as a PROM (premature rupture of the membranes), and it's one diary date you can do without. Your doctor will use a strip of litmus paper to check that it is amniotic fluid and that you haven't just peed yourself. (Pee is acidic and amniotic fluid is alkaline.)

If it is a PROM, you and your baby will be watched more closely than a New Hampshire primary, because premature labor, infection, and fetal distress are all distinct possibilities. Your dates, and the extent of the leak, will determine your options. The whole drama will be played out in the hospital, because not only is fluid coming out, but bacteria could be getting in. Cervical swabs will be taken to see if they produce anything nasty in the lab. They will also provide clues on the best antibiotics with which to hit back. A lot of doctors won't wait for the results, and will pump you full of broad spectrum antibiotics, which are the Green Berets of bacterial warfare. Depending on timetables, both you and your baby may also need antibiotics after the delivery. This can be really tough emotionally because babies get their dose via injection and there's absolutely no truth in the line that some doctors come out with—namely, that newborn babies don't feel pain. Overkill is often the object of the exercise, so don't be surprised if you start smelling the antibiotics as they seep out of your skin.

Speaking of smell, you might hear medical staff talking about the smell of the "liquor," which is what doctors sometimes call amniotic fluid (heaven knows why, because you'd never serve it on the rocks). The smell's important: if it's really whiffy—and you don't have to be an expert to notice— it's a sign of infection. Another bad sign is meconium in the fluid, which means that your baby's so scared that it's shitting itself, and has dumped some of the sticky black poop that it's supposed to hang on to until it's born.

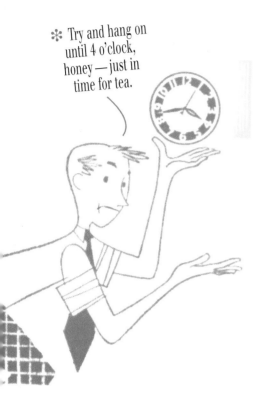

Try and hang on until 4 o'clock, honey—just in time for tea.

It's all in the timing

If you spring a leak before about 33 or 34 weeks, when the finishing touches to the lungs take place, your physician may try to buy time by using antibiotics to fight any infection, insisting on bed rest, and using drugs to stall contractions and steroids to speed up bumpsie's development. Most babies will need extra help at this stage, because they don't have enough surfactant, which is the slimy coating that stops the lungs sticking together during the first few breaths. If you've reached 33 or 34 weeks, and the baby is vertex (headfirst), your doctor may suggest delivery.

Another problem with PROMs is that the umbilical cord can be swept down into the cervical opening, or into the vagina itself. The earlier the leak, the bigger the risk, because there's more room for the cord to whoosh past the baby. Any pressure on the cord could put the squeeze on baby's oxygen supply, so an emergency Cesarean is almost inevitable. In the meantime, you might be asked to kneel down, doggy style, with your butt in the air. Not comfortable, but it should make the baby slide forward and away from the cord.

How early is early?

In most states bumpsie is considered "viable" after 24 weeks, but that's a legal definition, not a medical one. The real world is a lot tougher, and the chances of a baby surviving if born before 24 weeks—which is where many other countries draw the line of "viability"—are still very, very slim. Many of those who do pull through will be left with serious disabilities. However, medical care is improving all the time, and some babies fight harder than Mike Tyson, so there are now a small but growing number of "micro-preterms" who were born before 24 weeks.

Babies born this early have a lot of problems. Their lungs aren't fully developed, and they have a bad habit of forgetting to breathe; heart problems are more common; their skull bones are still quite soft, so if the

---

FISHY FACT

Fish oil capsules, rich in Omega-3 fatty acids, have been shown to decrease premature labor rates. These fatty acids are also found in salmon, herring, and other fish (12 ounces of fish a week is the current recommendation, but not from local waters). See page 23 for fish to avoid during pregnancy.

ESSENTIALS

EARLY ARRIVALS—WHAT HAPPENS

I used to be a two-pound weakling!

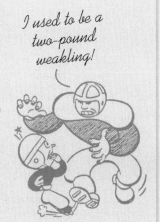

Babies who arrive early, or with more drama than a daytime soap opera, are usually rushed straight to the neonatal intensive care unit (NICU) or special care baby unit (SCBU), which can be really tough on the new parents. It's not always possible to hold the baby at first, and he or she might have to stay in a humidi-crib, hooked up to an artificial respirator and IV lines. However, physical contact is encouraged, and many units now use kangaroo care (skin to skin contact and cuddling). Doctors tend to be cautious when they esti-mate for how long babies will need special care, so don't be too downhearted at initial estimates: they can shrink. Another reas-suring thing about having a baby in the NICU or SCBU is that you'll discover how many people you know—often guys who are built like quarterbacks—who were born early.

baby's head is squashed and squeezed during delivery, there is a risk of brain damage caused by bleeding in the fragile head; they haven't learned how to suck, and have to be fed by tubes; they're not very good at keeping warm, and lose heat more quickly because they don't have much body fat; and they often get jaundice, which makes them look like they've been using a cheap fake tan, and can cause liver and hearing damage.

Every extra day on the inside, and every extra ounce (25 g) of weight, is a bonus, so the longer your bun can be kept in the oven, the better its chances. Size matters, but gestational age is still more important in lung development and bowel maturity. Steroids given to the mother help to improve the chances of lung maturity and are used whenever possible. Not that long ago, it was touch and go for babies of 30 and 32 weeks, but now they have pretty much the same prospects as those who've gone for the full count, and some may even be larger than fullterm babies who are small for their dates. A baby born six weeks early weighing 5 pounds, 8 ounces (2.5 kg)—which is on a real "Ouch!" trajectory, if you follow the centile charts—might have fewer problems than a very small baby who arrives on time.

✳ Felicity's tip is to try and keep your bun in the oven for as long as the recipe requires.

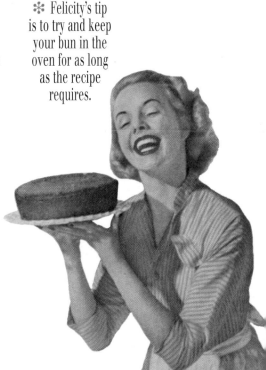

LAST-MINUTE PLANNING

Most babies stick more or less to the schedule, so the last few weeks usually provide plenty of time for last-minute planning. This allows you to make sure that your urban warrior's survival skills are up to scratch, and that he knows how all the household appliances work. If you lay the groundwork now, it will make life a lot easier during the first few weeks with a new baby, when you might be so tired that you can't think straight, and the simplest outing can turn into a military operation.

LOST BAGGAGE

Leave the Louis Vuittons at home —unless they're a cheap knock-off. Good baggage and jewelry are more trouble than they're worth when you're in the hospital. Most medical centers warn that they won't be held responsible for theft and damage.

❋ Cute! Matching mom and baby baggage for the trip of a lifetime!

Get the car serviced, make sure it's always full of gas, and organize a Plan B if your partner's not around to drive you: don't even think about driving yourself when you're in labor. If you live some distance from the hospital or birth center, time the journey during rush hour and at a quiet time so that you have a clear idea of how long to leave at any time of day or night. Look out for advance warnings of roadworks along the route, and investigate alternatives. If you have older children and don't plan to have them at the birth, make arrangements for a friend or family member to look after them when the action starts. Be sure to buy them a present from the new baby to head off any envy or sibling rivalry: this can be wrapped and put in your hospital bag.

Cook and freeze as much food as you can: your partner will appreciate being able to grab something quickly, and having a stash of homemade soups, pasta sauces, and casseroles will make it a lot easier to get through the first week or so at home. Stock up on dried foods, such as rice and pasta, as well as household cleaning stuff. Speaking of which, if you don't have one, it's worth trying to find a cleaner or booking one through an agency, even if it's only for a week or two.

Pack an overnight bag with all the things you're likely to need in the hospital. Include a few cotton nightdresses that button down the front and have short, or very loose, sleeves: this is useful for breast-feeding and blood pressure checks. Pack plenty of cotton briefs, and a supply of absorbent sanitary pads. You'll need at least two or three supportive nursing bras (cotton ones are best), and a supply of absorbent breast pads to soak up any leaks. You'll need a few bits of loose, comfortable clothing to wear around the ward during the day, and something to travel home in, plus a pair of slippers or slip-on shoes. A lipstick and mascara will make it easier to look back on those early photos of you and the baby without cringing. For the baby, pack a few singlets and jumpsuits, scratch mittens, a hat, and diapers. It's also a good idea to take along at least one of your own baby blankets or shawls so that you can wrap the baby in something familiar for the journey home. Some hospitals also expect you to take your own pillow, which is usually more comfortable than hospital pillows anyway.

Don't forget to include birth aids such as TENS machines, music cassette tapes or CDs, and food and drink for your birth partner. Include a few glucose candies for yourself in case it's a long delivery, and some nutritious snacks (such as crispbread, nuts, or dried fruit) to prevent snack attacks during midnight breast-feeding sessions. You might also want to include: a water spray to keep you cool in labor; scent or aromatherapy oils to block out the hospital smell; massage balls or rollers; and lip balm and moisturizer. Don't forget your usual toiletries. Draw up a list of telephone numbers for those people who will need to be informed of the birth. Take coins or a card to pay for the calls (no cell phones allowed in the hospital). You could prepare a telephone tree, in which you call one or two people and they call one or two other people in turn, and so on. You can also take a book or a couple of magazines (you wish!), and a notebook and pen to jot down things that you need to remember. Rather like your stomach muscles, your short-term memory won't bounce back right away.

✳ Great! Looks as if I'll have time to change my cravat before D-day!

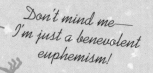

*Don't mind me—
I'm just a benevolent
euphemism!*

Labor
when push comes to SHOVE   OUCH!!!

verage" and "labor" are like "designer" and "bargain": two words that don't belong in the same sentence. For starters, a lot depends on when you start counting. Labor's a bit like being a teenager. There are phases that we've all gotta go through, but we all go through them at our own pace. Some girls are destined to be prom queens, while others seem to get every zit and every bit of boy trouble going.

❋ *Having a baby is as simple as 1 2 3, Cecil. First you go to the hospital...*

Officially, there are three stages. The first stage usually lasts around 12 hours if you haven't had a baby before, and about six hours if your equipment has already been tested—at least, that's what the textbooks say. The easy part within the first stage—relatively, that is—is the "latent" phase. It takes around six to eight hours, and by the end of it your cervix will be 3–4 cm dilated. Then you step up a gear into the "active" phase, when contractions get more serious and come more often. This means that it's time to get to the hospital. This stage lasts until you're fully dilated—a perfect 10 cm—and can last another four to six hours. The last little bit of the first stage is sometimes known as "transition"—the head may be descending at this point and the contractions may be more painful and close together. It's really quick, but sometimes it's also really weird (*see pages 180–185*).

The second stage of labor is when push comes to shove, and you have to work with the contractions to squeeze your baby out. The first time around, it usually takes around two hours, but with subsequent babies your nurse-midwife may need a catcher's mitt, because it can go much more quickly—and once you've discovered which buttons and muscles to push, you really can PUSH!

The third stage is when the placenta is expelled. This can be spontaneously expelled, which can take a few minutes or more, or gentle assisted traction (steady pulling) can expedite delivery. In very rare cases, a manual extraction has to be performed. After the placenta is delivered, It's common practice to give moms a shot of Pitocin (oxytocin), or add it to their IV, to reduce blood loss by helping uterine contractions.

That's the rough guide to giving birth, but as the next pages show, no two deliveries are ever the same, not even when you're doing it second or third time around.

Sometimes the first stage action starts with your waters breaking and a whoosh of fluid that looks like pee and soaks your shoes. Even if you can keep your balance on Blahniks at this stage, it's best not to risk it! You might get a slow buildup involving a squeezing sensation around your belly, or a dull ache in the small of your back. Some women experience a pulling sensation at the tops of the thighs. Another unmistakable sign that bumpsie is about to drop is finding a little glob of stuff like thick jelly in your pants. You might also get a "show." This has nothing to do with feathers and Elvis impersonators: it's a little bit of mucus and blood that shows that your cervix is limbering up for the big stretch. We also have a new wives' tale to throw into the ocean of superstition that surrounds having children: every pregnancy involves a certain amount of pain and difficulty, so if you've had a really shitty pregnancy you may have a breeze of a birth, but if you've sailed through pregnancy, don't assume that it will be just as simple once the time comes to deliver the goods. There are no rules, so it helps to expect the unexpected.

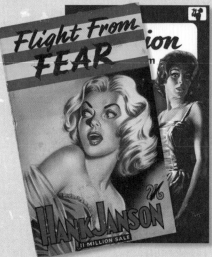

✻ ...then you do the scary bit, with the screaming and pain...

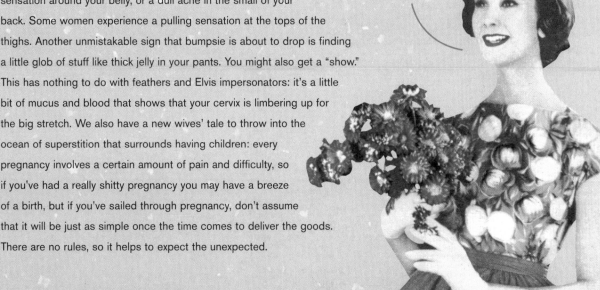

✻ ... and then people give you lots of lovely flowers!

HARD LABOR?

" I was getting out of the car when I felt a dribble in my panties, and by the time I stood up, this pale yellow liquid was gushing down my legs. You didn't have to be Einstein to work out what was happening. I drove home in a panic. My shoes were soaked, and they kept slipping off the accelerator and brake pedals. Looking back, I should have called Mark and got him to pick me up. By the time I got home, the contractions had started, and they were already about 12 minutes apart when Mark arrived. I was getting really panicky that we wouldn't make it to the hospital in time. What a joke! The contractions went on like that for another six hours before the nurse-midwife finally said I was 3 cm dilated. Yippee, we'd made it to first base! "

KAREN, 31

" My panties had felt a bit wet the day before, and then I noticed a bit of blood in this gluey goop. I rang a friend who'd just had a baby, and she thought it was probably a "show." Heaven knows why, but I put it in a jar in the refrigerator in case the doctor wanted to see it. It was almost two full days later that I started to get this heavy feeling around my back, and shooting pains on the inside of my legs. I rang Jenny again, and she said that the back bit could be labor pains, but she hadn't felt anything at all in her legs, so I decided to sit it out. Over the next ten hours, the pains in my legs went away, but the ache in my back got worse. That night I couldn't sleep at all and was getting really fed up. I began to think they could be contractions, but both Jenny and the doctor had said that real contractions would keep getting worse, and these just seemed to stay the same—painful, but not too bad. By the next morning I'd really had enough, and called the hospital to say we were on our way there. I figured I'd talk them into inducing me. I just wanted that baby out, now! There was no need: I had started to dilate—just—and because I was so tired, they started a Pitocin infusion to speed things up. That helped, but it was still another 13 hours before I was holding my baby. I figure it must be some sort of record: counting from the 'show,' I was in labor for almost four days! "

MADELEINE, 24

Hey, moms, when the going gets tough...

“ At first I wasn't really sure. I had this dull ache in the small of my back, and every so often it got a bit crampy, like period pains. Around 3:00 p.m. I started getting the runs really badly, and I must have spent the next half-hour in the bathroom, shitting and peeing at the same time. Once everything was out of my system, it eased off a bit and I fell asleep. Then the pains came back with a vengeance, but I still wasn't convinced I was in labor: I hadn't had a show, I still had a week to go, and the pains didn't seem to follow any pattern. Bill insisted we call the doctor, and she suggested that I should go in. I was already 2 cm dilated and Matthew was born 10 hours later. ”   CELIA, 38

“ By the time I did actually go into labor, I don't know who was more relieved, me or my nurse-midwife. I'd had strong Braxton Hicks contractions from 34 weeks, but in the final couple of weeks they got a lot worse. The first false alarm came at 38 weeks. I noticed a bit of brownish blood on the sheets, and an hour or so later I started getting strong contractions every ten minutes. But when we got to the hospital the nurse-midwife said my cervix was rock hard and shut tight, and the blood was because of an internal examination the day before. I felt a complete klutz, but nowhere near as dumb as I did after false alarm number four. What was really funny was that when the action did start, I knew, absolutely for certain, what it was. ”   LETITIA, 27

....remember it's me you're playing for.

“ All day I'd been feeling edgy, pacing around checking things. Peter thought I was mad when I suggested calling the doctor again. I still had six weeks to go, and had already insisted on seeing him twice that week because—well, just because. He couldn't find anything wrong, and it wasn't as if there was anything specific I could tell him. I just had this gut feeling that something was going to happen. In the end, I convinced Peter to drive me to the birth center: he figured it was the only way to shut me up. I was having contractions by the time we got there, and 90 minutes later I was holding my baby. If it hadn't been my second child I don't think I'd have been so insistent. ”   JODIE, 37

THE FINAL COUNTDOWN AND SHE'S OFF!

If you're a first-timer, one clue that you will appreciate is the baby's "engagement." This is a happy occasion: the baby's head slips down into your pelvis, giving you a break from indigestion, heartburn, and pain around the rib cage. Engagement changes the shape of your bump and women describe it as like having a shelf on the upper abdomen as the baby's head drops down into the pelvis! On the down side, it may also mean that bumpsie's head will press on your bladder, making you pee constantly.

❊ And when I've finished sandblasting the dinner plates, I'm going to varnish the dog.

Once the engagement's been announced, your walking style will look like a cross between a sluggish penguin and John Wayne after a long day in the saddle. If it's your first baby, engagement will happen two to four weeks before D-day. If it doesn't, your physician or nurse-midwife will reassess the size of the baby, its position, and the size of your pelvis, giving you a fair idea of what to expect during labor. For old hands, the head probably won't get engaged until labor's actually started.

A day or two before the action starts, some women get a surge of energy. You might be overtaken by an urgent desire to clean the entire house. Don't do it! Resist the temptation to do anything more strenuous than checking that your bag is packed; you're going to need all the energy you can get once labor starts. Some people call this energy rush the "nesting instinct," and there is something quite basic and animal about it, as if some sort of primitive programming is kicking in. This energy surge can happen when babies decide to ignore the schedule and turn up early. We've known moms who rushed out to buy baby equipment and clothing a day or two before giving birth five or six weeks early, so if you are getting twitchy, trust your instincts.

Babies' movements change during the last weeks—with less room, the movements are less dramatic but should be plentiful. There's an old wives' tale that they become a lot quieter just before contractions start, and a lot of moms swear that this is true, but a lot of doctors say it's dangerous to think in these terms, because a lack of movement can also mean that something's wrong. If you're worried, lie on your side, counting movements, preferably after a sweet drink or light snack. Most moms will log ten movements within an hour. If you get to two hours and still haven't felt ten squirms, wriggles, or whatever, get medical advice.

Your vagina may feel very wet, and there's often a great deal of mucus that feels thicker than usual. Don't panic if you see little bits of blood, or if this "mom-juice" is a pinkish color: this just means that it's showtime, and the curtain's going up! As mentioned previously, the "show" can appear when your cervix begins to thin out and stretch, popping a few little blood vessels along the way. This sort of show should always be a bit off-Broadway, small and intimate. Anything resembling a period or serious bleeding needs urgent investigation. The show usually means that labor will start within a day, but it can take longer. If your show is more brown than red in color, then it's probably not a show at all, but just a dress rehearsal. This is most likely to happen if you've had an internal examination recently.

Pooping and peeing even more than usual (yes, it really is possible!) are sure signs that something's about to happen. A day or two before going into labor, your uterus starts pumping out prostaglandin, a hormone that gives you the shits. At first you just need to go a lot more, and when you're close to kick off, the poop often gets loose, too.

Before going into labor, some women shake and shiver so much that you'd think they had shoved a finger in a power socket. It doesn't necessarily mean that they're terrified of going into labor, although it can be pretty scary when it starts to happen. It's the body's way of getting rid of tension, and it's most likely to happen if you're really wound up and anxious.

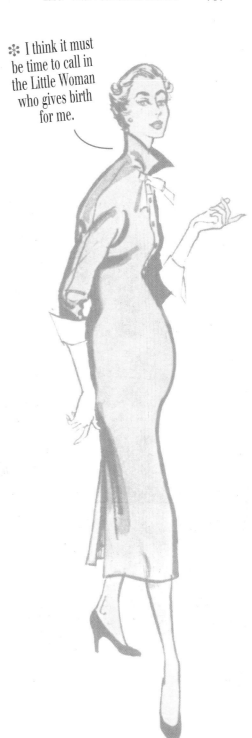

✻ I think it must be time to call in the Little Woman who gives birth for me.

✳ Red Leader to Braxton Hicks: time to scramble, over and out.

False alarms

Braxton Hicks contractions are the biggest cause of false alarms, and no wonder. Some women get some real gut crunchers that leave them doubled up with pain and gasping for breath, while others can be in the early stages of labor and still feel little more than a bit of tightness around their back and belly. That's why the early action is called the "latent" phase—contractions can be so mild that you don't even notice them.

So how do you tell the difference between early labor and Braxton Hicks? There are no hard-and-fast rules, but if the contractions ease up, or stop completely when you walk around or change position, then they're probably Braxton Hicks. Real contractions tend to spread out from your lower back, while Braxton Hicks are more likely to start in your belly or crotch.

The most obvious difference between Braxton Hicks and real labor is that real labor doesn't go away, and the contractions get stronger and more frequent. However, don't be blindsided by all that stuff in the movies about timing your contractions. Yes, the majority of women do get a reasonably steady buildup, and your doctor will probably suggest calling when your contractions come at certain intervals (anything from five to ten minutes apart, depending on how far away from the hospital you live). However, you shouldn't wait until every single contraction is coming on cue: it might never happen. Some women are well into active labor, or even the second stage, before their contractions slip into anything resembling a regular pattern.

Real contractions are quite short at first, lasting for a minute at most, and tend to come at regular intervals. They usually hurt and often come with backache. Your belly will tighten up and get hard while they're going on. Braxton Hicks contractions are much more erratic,

ESSENTIALS

PERFECT PLANNING

You might have covered every contingency like the books say you should. The perfect plan goes something like this. You had the car fully serviced weeks ago. It's never had less than half a tank of gas for the past two months. Your partner has timed the journey to the hospital down to the last second, and double-checked that there aren't any roadworks along the way. There's a pillow and blanket so that you can keep warm and comfy while stretching out on the back seat. You've already worked out how to fasten the seatbelt loosely under your belly. Your partner knows which hospital entrance to drop you off at, and the quickest route to the long-term parking lot. He's either paid for this in advance, or has enough coins in the glove compartment to buy a 24-hour ticket. You've preregistered at the hospital and they've got all your health insurance details, so there's almost no paperwork left to do. You've got all the time in the world to slip into your favorite nightdress, rearrange the furniture for optimal feng shui, and admire the flock of pigs that's flying past the labor room window.

and they may be short. There's never any backache, and sometimes the contractions themselves don't hurt either. If in doubt, call your doctor or birth center. These guys are used to working all hours of the night and day, and are always there to help. But perhaps the most convincing of all is that little inner voice—and who knows whether it's your's or the kid's—that screams "IT'S TIME!"

Getting to the hospital

If you're told that it's time to go to the hospital, then the first thing to do is to stay calm. You should still have plenty of time to get there. If you have any doubts about the reliability of your car or the route to the hospital, call a cab (particularly if parking at the hospital is a pain in the neck as well as a pain in the pocket). Either way, take your cell phone with you so that you can call for help on the way if you think you're not going to make it. First-time moms are highly unlikely to get caught out, but the more babies you have, the quicker they come out and the better your body gets at pushing, even when you don't want to do so (see page 160).

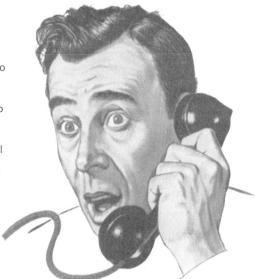

❄ Can you hold on a little longer sweet pea? The game'll be over in fifteen.

LET THE LABOR BEGIN AND THE PANTING START

Once you get to the hospital, or once your delivery person gets to you if it's a home birth, the nurse-midwife will make a note of any relevant medical information or special needs (medical ones, not the "hold the mayo" variety), and will probably ask you to sign some routine consent forms. You'll have a quick checkup, which should include peeing in yet another jar, having your blood pressure, temperature, and pulse taken, and an internal examination.

The internal is done to see how dilated and effaced your cervix is and the position and station of the baby (where baby is in relation to your pelvic bones). Don't worry, no one's going to stick a ruler up there: two fingers do the job. The width of the forefinger and middle finger together is about 3 cm, the magic milestone that marks the start of the second phase.

In many hospitals, shaving has—as we've already discussed—gone the way of big shoulder pads and Lycra leggings. If yours is stuck in a timewarp and you don't want it, say so! Shaving is only done before a C-section along the bikini line. A lot of hospitals will want to put in an IV line. While all of this is going on, it's a good idea for your partner to grab a snack, and make a few calls to let people know you're on the launch pad and counting down.

✳ You have to be two fingers dilated, lady, that's TWO fingers.

Babe watch

Once the preliminaries have been done, most moms-in-the-making are hooked up to a monitor that prints out two zig-zaggy graphs, rather like a lie detector (although this one can tell fibs: see opposite). Most monitors have a wide strap that goes around your tummy, making you look like a giant hard-boiled egg with an anchovy on top, very attractive. But hey, don't worry: any shred of dignity that you had left was checked in at the admissions desk. The main unit of the monitor records your contractions and your baby's heartbeat. Strap-on monitors tend to go berserk when you move around, so you'll be asked to stay as still as possible. This is easier said than done when your womb is doing more muscle-flexing than Jean Claude van Damme. Don't panic if they can't find a heartbeat at first: it's usually the result of extra padding (too many Oreos and ice cream, perhaps) or the baby being curled up in a funny position. In a year or three, you'll call this sort of game "Pin the Tail on the Donkey."

Comparing the two graphs gives a pretty good idea of how your baby's doing, and if it's OK you could be off the monitor in 20 or 30 minutes. If you're not, ask why. In theory, continuous monitoring provides early warnings of any problems. In practice, it can make mountains out of molehills, making the medical staff jumpy, and you're much more likely to experience some sort of intervention such as vacuum delivery, forceps, or a C-section. However, continuous monitoring is advisable in high-risk pregnancies. It is also a good idea to follow the guidelines for intermittent monitoring during active labor if there isn't one-on-one nursing staff. In early labor, if you have to be in the hospital after the initial monitoring, you can walk around and check the fetal heart rate intermittently.

Another good reason to get up and off your back is that it really pays to be an upright citizen. Standing or squatting will push the weight of your baby down onto your cervix, adding extra value to every contraction. This can make the difference between a comfortable middle distance run and a hard marathon. Other positions that beat lying on your back and thinking, "Who the hell got me into this?", include: kneeling forward with your partner supporting your weight; sitting astride a chair and leaning on the back; and leaning onto a wall or desk. If you're getting a lot of pain in your back (some people call this back labor), try going down onto all fours, doggy style, and stick your butt in the air. It may not be the best option for family photos, but it works in this context.

KNOW THE JARGON

When it comes to your cervix, these words will be coming thicker and faster than your contractions. "Effacement" refers to the thinning out of the cervix in preparation for the birth and "dilation" refers to how open it is.

✳ Time to get on all fours, I just can't hold on any longer...

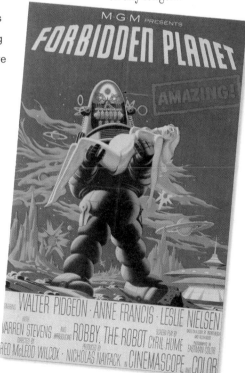

SCHEDULES AND INDUCTION

Babies are like house guests: it's great when they arrive, but sometimes they need a nudge to let them know it's time to leave. This is called induction, which also happens to army recruits. Maybe that's why many moms-to-be find it scary. There are a number of reasons for inducing babies. Good ones include certain conditions that affect the mother's health, such as pre-eclampsia and diabetes, or risks to the baby's well-being such as stalled growth, and being more overdue than a forgotten library book.

Lousy reasons include fitting delivery around your doctor's golf schedule, or trying to achieve a particular astrological alignment. Gray areas might be if you have to schedule childcare or live far from the hospital or are anxious because of a previous difficult delivery. Induction is relatively safe and straightforward, but it should never be done for personal convenience, no matter who the person is. It pays to respect your cervical ripening before electively inducing and to make sure that the baby is really fullterm.

Who's counting?

All due dates are guesstimates and, just like dress sizes, some are more accurate than others. Technically, two weeks either side of the due date is "on time," and some poor women drag it out until 44 weeks. By that time we'd want the baby dragged out, even if it is kicking and screaming. Most doctors and hospitals start getting edgy after a week, and suggest induction after two. Some will cut you a little more slack, particularly if the baby's OK, and ultrasound and other tests suggest that the problem is with your dates rather than your dispatch system. A quick but accurate guide to dating is to check the timing of physical milestones along the way, such as early HCG levels, transvaginal ultrasound in the first trimester, the first time the fetal heart could be heard, first movements, and the fundus measurements (which

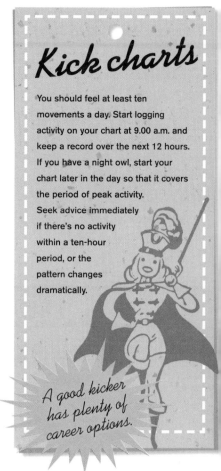

Kick charts

You should feel at least ten movements a day. Start logging activity on your chart at 9.00 a.m. and keep a record over the next 12 hours. If you have a night owl, start your chart later in the day so that it covers the period of peak activity. Seek advice immediately if there's no activity within a ten-hour period, or the pattern changes dramatically.

A good kicker has plenty of career options.

You want me to do WHAT with these hot towels?

show how high up your uterus is getting). If these all tally, your dates are probably right and you will be induced. Sometimes, in cases of an indicated induction before 39 weeks (for maternal or fetal indications), which is not immediately urgent, an amniocentesis may be carried out to test the fluid for markers that the baby's lungs are mature.

Pregnancy can sometimes continue quite happily (for Junior at least) into the tenth month, but the longer it lasts, the greater the risk that your placenta will pack up. Also, your baby might get too big to squeeze through your pelvis. Checks to ensure that the baby's OK include: kick charts; the non-stress test (a fancy name for comparing the fetal heartrate with fetal movements); and fetal acoustical stimulation (FAS, which basically involves ringing the doorbell to see if anyone's moving about inside). There is also something called the oxytocin challenge test, which is done less frequently. This is done with a Pitocin pump giving you several contractions and making sure the fetal heart rate remains stable. You could also be given a shot of oxytocin. Either way, the fetus is monitored to see how it reacts to this chemical dig in the ribs, and you get the fun of a few practice contractions. Then there's a biophysical profile (BPP), which is an ultrasound-derived examination with the nonstress test thrown in. A high score on this test means that the placenta is functioning well and that there is no cause for immediate action.

Ripe for the plucking

The first step is to find out how ripe your cervix is. Yes, we're back to the fruit fetishes again. Just like you'd do with an avocado, your nurse-midwife gives your cervix a gentle squeeze to see if it's starting to soften, or is still rock hard and a million miles from making guacamole. The nurse-midwife examines the cervix and checks its position, consistency, and effacement. The baby's

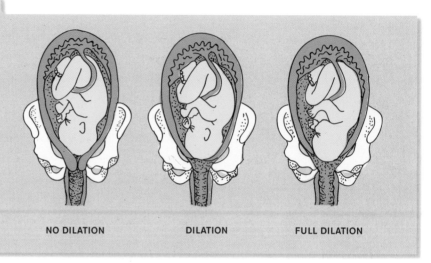

ESSENTIALS

DILATION

During the first stage of labor (the latent phase), the cervix starts to efface (thin out) and dilates (opens) to around 3 cm. Then it continues to dilate between 1 and 1.5 cm every hour during the active phase until it reaches 10 cm (complete dilation).

NO DILATION   **DILATION**   **FULL DILATION**

✳ Larry soon realized that walking in circles was not going to help.

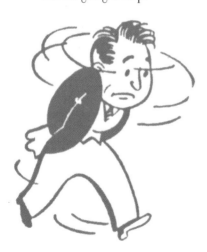

head is also checked with respect to the maternal pelvic bones. The result is given as a Bishop score (which sounds like a goal for the Vatican Red Sox—or would they be Purple Sox?). This is your inducibility rating, and five different factors are given a rating from zero to three. A soft, shortened cervix that's already started to open scores highly, particularly if the baby's head is already well down into your pelvis, and your cervix is pointing forward, not toward your butt. You'll get nil points for one that's still firm, shows no signs of opening, and hasn't begun to shorten. A Bishop score of six or more means there's a good chance that induction will work.

There are two ways to get things moving. One uses medication such as prostaglandins and Pitocin, and this is usually accompanied by an amniotomy (breaking the amniotic sac with something that looks like a crochet hook). If you've got a Bishop score of five or less (meaning that your cervix is not soft or thinned out or dilated, and that the baby's presenting part is high), your cervix will need a little artificial ripening. This is done with prostaglandins by gel or suppositories or tablets placed vaginally or even with a foley catheter in the cervix (a foley catheter is usually used to drain the bladder, but it can be used to mechanically dilate the cervix). This may be repeated every three or four hours. Many women believe that induced labor is more painful—hey, active labor is painful and that is the point of induction—to get you into active labor.

If the cervix is open enough, the baby's membranes will be ruptured, and you'll be put on an IV of oxytocin, usually controlled carefully with a pump, in order to activate contractions. (In some hospitals and birth centers they call it Pitocin, which is the brand name.) Oxytocin is produced in increasing amounts throughout the pregnancy, but it doesn't really kick in and start contractions until levels of other hormones drop, just before the start of labor. The drip rate of oxytocin is steadily increased until you get 45-second contractions every three minutes. There's no set dosage, as some women are more sensitive to oxytocin than others. If you are given too much, the effect of the medication is so shortlived that turning off the oxytocin drip will eliminate its effect.

✳ A keen supporter of active childbirth, Greg offered to burst the amniotic sac himself.

By hook or by hook

"Amniotomy" is doctor speak for bursting baby's bubble. The amniotic sac is punctured with an instrument called an amnihook, which is a glorified crochet hook. If it's gotta be done, it's gotta be done. You will be asked to have a pee first, just to make sure that there's nothing in your bladder that will slow up the action, and in case you pee yourself anyway with…let's call it excitement. Your doctor or nurse-midwife will also want a good look at the amniotic fluid to check for meconium. There's a sudden whoosh of fluid, which is often closely followed by contractions. If the amniotic sac has been overfilled, small amounts of fluid called "polyhydramnios" may be siphoned off gradually using a long needle. This avoids a sudden surge, which could push the umbilical cord out of the cervix or dislodge the placenta.

ACTIVE SERVICE   GET MOVING!

I t usually takes a first-timer between six and eight hours to get to the 3-cm dilation stage, which makes the average snail look like Carl Lewis. Unless you're incredibly unlucky, or have the pain threshold of a gnat, this first bit is usually easily manageable, and unless there is a high-risk situation, you're better off at home, walking around. In fact, it's so easy that some women don't even notice it, or are aware of nothing more than a vague sense of tension around the belly.

Houston, Houston do you read? Request decoder for TENS machine.

If you're using a TENS machine, have a shower during this phase and ask someone to help you put it on. Once the unit's on, you have to stay dry, because water and electricity are not a brilliant combination. Ignore anyone who says it's too early and that you don't need it yet: they don't know what they're talking about. TENS works on a slow buildup, so if you wait until you're actually finding contractions uncomfortable, it won't be anywhere near as effective. Putting it on early gives your body a chance to start producing more endorphins and dispatching them to the right nerve junctions. It also gives you plenty of time to get the hang of the controls—not that it's rocket science.

This is also the time to try visualization, if that's your thing. Don't be too tough on yourself if you get the giggles; quite frankly, some of the suggestions we've heard from birth coaches can be laughable. One of our favorites is: "Now, picture your cervix as a delicate pink rosebud, its petals damp with dew. Slowly allow the petals to unfurl, gently opening their faces to the sun so that your little flower fairy can fly free..." Sorry, but we just couldn't convince ourselves that the sun really did shine out of our muff, and we figured that anyone who called bumpsie a flower fairy was probably away with the fairies themselves. Thanks, but no thanks. That said, these gentler contractions do give you a chance to practice breathing and to try adopting a Zenlike calm. The longer that you tell yourself you're coping well, the longer you will cope well.

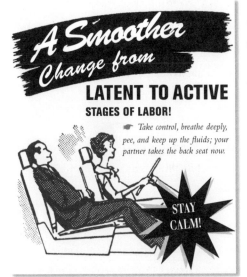

A Smoother Change from LATENT TO ACTIVE STAGES OF LABOR!

☞ *Take control, breathe deeply, pee, and keep up the fluids; your partner takes the back seat now.*

STAY CALM!

Gear shift

Generally, once you've reached the more active phase, you should dilate between 1 cm and 1.5 cm every hour. Contractions come more quickly—every two or three minutes—and will last for up to a minute. If the amniotic sac is still intact, it should rupture anytime now, or be ruptured by your nurse-midwife or physician. Try to remember to have a pee: the nerve endings down there are in such a spin that you may not notice that you need to go. Deep breathing will help to keep you calm and ensure that there's plenty of oxygen floating around your system and getting to the baby. It's also important to stay hydrated by sucking ice cubes or taking sips of water. Some birth centers try to restrict your fluids in case there is an emergency and you need a general anesthetic.

For most women the last few centimeters of dilation are the toughest bit of childbirth, because the contractions are strong and painful and seem to come almost on top of each other, but you don't yet have the distraction and focus of actively pushing. There's a lot going on down there. During this phase, the cervix is effacing (or thinning out), and dilating, and the fetal presenting part is descending. The chances are you're getting tired, fed up, and perhaps even a bit frightened.

Stay focused on your goal, as one of those motivational speakers would say. Try out different positions: you'll probably find that a lot of them come instinctively, like rocking back and forth on all fours. By this time, a lot of women find that squatting makes contractions too intense for comfort, but it might help to slip down into a squat between contractions, and then stand up when things start tightening up again. You may look like a jack in the box that's blown a fuse, but who cares? It doesn't matter a damn what you look like. If it's comfortable, do it.

TIME WARP

Try not to be a clock-watcher—you've probably already worked out that it's rarely a good career move, but it can be an even worse one when you're having a baby. Your sense of time becomes totally skewed when you're in labor, stretching seconds or wiping entire hours, but watching the clock can also skew your experience of labor and make moments seem like a marathon.

PAIN, PAIN, GO AWAY

As the pace picks up you may want to scream, "GIMME DRUGS! NOW!" or just scream, period. Feel free, particularly if this stage goes on for a long time. You are the only one who really knows how bad or how bearable the pain really is, and they don't give out medals for going cold turkey. If you have to deal later on with one of those sanctimonious types who believes that there's some sort of virtue in putting yourself through utter agony, just tell them you got through with meditation and aromatherapy.

If, on the other hand, the sanctimonious type is your birth partner, try hitting them very hard. Explain that this displacement activity is the only way that you're going to get through. It's amazing how a little pain can change someone's attitude to pain relief.

Generally speaking, you call the shots, but occasionally women ask for pain relief and then start to suspect that their nurse-midwife is stalling. You may not want to hear this, but she probably is, and although you probably won't think so at the time, she's actually doing you a favor. It's all down to timing. If you're really close to being fully dilated—and the nurse-midwife or physician is the only one who can see what's going on down there—you could be through this last tricky bit, and on the home stretch, by the time the anesthetist arrives on the ward and puts in the plumbing for an epidural. There's also a danger that if you give painkillers, such as Demerol, at this relatively late stage, the baby will be drowsy and lazy about breathing and sucking when it comes out. "See if you can manage another 20 minutes," is the mantra of most delivery people at this point of the labor.

It's a difficult balancing act, and the best way to get it right is to communicate as much information as possible to your nurse-midwife. Tell her if the pain is really unbearable, but also be prepared to listen, and believe her, if she says you're doing really well and the worst of it is nearly over. Think about each contraction as being one less rather than

Painkillers! Now! Or I'll ram your speculum where the sun don't shine!

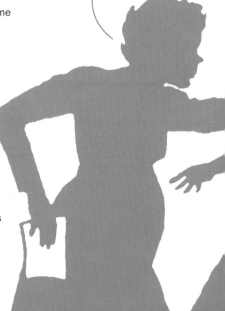

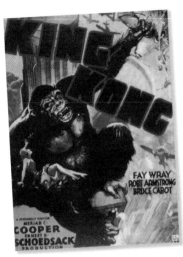

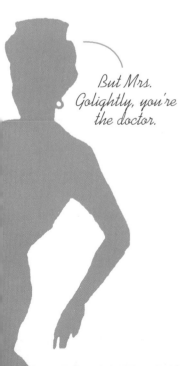

✳ Sometimes only the Fay Wray option will do. Scream — long and loud.

But Mrs. Golightly, you're the doctor.

one more, and make the most of the little breaks in between. Try to relax between contractions. OK, we know that's a lot easier said than done, but it will help to conserve your energy and give your body a chance to go with the flow. Getting all scrunched up and tense is more likely to slow things down and make the pain seem even worse.

Go slow

Dilation that's any slower than 1 cm per hour is considered abnormal. In reality, though, contractions can still be pretty erratic at this point, and something as simple as changing positions can change the pace dramatically. Policies vary, but so long as your contractions don't grind to a complete halt, and both you and your baby are OK, your nurse-midwife or physician might cut you a bit of slack. We're all different. Some women begin really slowly and then sprint to the finish line, while others start with a surge and then seem to get stuck somewhere along the way. Your progress will be charted. If it falls too far behind, your physician or nurse-midwife may want to put their foot on the accelerator with a drip of oxytocin. This is sometimes called "active management of labor," and the aim is to ensure progressive dilation and descent of the baby within a certain time frame (usually between 12 and 18 hours after regular contractions begin) to decrease complications.

If you've reached full dilation, if the baby's head or presenting part is descending into the bony part of the pelvis, into what is known as "+2 station" (a number given in relation to the pelvic bones—0 is at the level of the spine, minus numbers are above this, and +5 is near delivery), and if the pelvis is deemed big enough, the doctor will attempt vacuum or forceps delivery. A lot of physicians and nurse-midwives would recommend one long before this point, particularly if it looks as though your baby may be too big, is in distress, or you're so exhausted that you're too bushed to push.

MAKING THE TRANSITION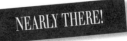

NEARLY THERE!

Just before the serious business of pushing starts, there's an interlude known as "transition," which can be one of the weirdest and most unsettling periods of the whole delivery. For some women, it's an almost religious experience. In a way, it is: it's a physical manifestation of the miracle of life, and women can be swept up into a state of euphoric bliss. Others talk about an overwhelming sense of release that is so intensely pleasurable, it's almost orgasmic. But a lot of women, me included, just lose it.

Lose what, you ask? Well, everything: your temper, humor, confidence, sense of time, patience, contact with reality, any semblance of control...in short, your marbles. Some women also lose the contents of their stomach, assuming there was anything left in there, or become unable to control their own body temperature. One minute you can be shivering uncontrollably with cold, and the next you can be soaked with sweat and hotter than the latest boy band.

✳ Buttoned-up cardigans prevent unnecessary behavior at this time, Sybil.

It's quite common to feel spaced out and confused. Even if you haven't had any medication, you may feel drugged. This is because there's so much oxygen being pumped down to the scene of the action that there may not be as much as usual getting to your brain. Sometimes there's such an overwhelming sense of momentous change taking place that women actually convince themselves they've given birth, and ask how come they didn't have to push. Tears of frustration or fury, or both, may suddenly overwhelm you. Even moms-in-the-making who've been coping incredibly well up to this point can suddenly be racked with doubts about their ability to cope. The massage and physical contact that was bliss a few minutes ago can suddenly become the most incredibly irritating intrusion into your personal space. Sponging your face with cool water sometimes helps, particularly if you're feeling really hot and hassled, but there are no guarantees. Clothing gets torn off, partners get chewed out, and life's a complete and utter bitch.

Transition usually lasts only a few minutes, although it can feel like a lifetime. Occasionally, it lasts for an hour or two. Apart from the moment when your baby actually comes out, it's the one point of the whole process that you and your birth partner are most likely to remember, if only because this is when you're most likely to suggest the surgical removal of his male parts to make sure that you're never in this position again. If he's not so lucky, you may even suggest ripping them off with your bare hands. Midwives and physicians come in for flak too, but don't worry, they don't take it personally. This may sound strangely masochistic, but it's a good sign, which means that the baby's well on its way. If you still have the energy for verbal abuse and a bit of primal screaming, you're in pretty good shape.

Sometimes there's not a lot your birth partner can do other than act as a verbal, and possibly physical, punchbag. There are times when a few words of calm encouragement can help the mom-in-the-making get through, but there are others when she'll just want everyone to shut the hell up. A birth partner should never, ever, *ever* say that they know how you feel. They haven't got a clue, not even if your partner's a woman who's had children before, because our brains quickly blur the memory. If they didn't, we'd have hit zero population growth a long time ago. One of the weird things about having a second or third child is that you often get to this point and suddenly think, "Oh shit, now I remember!"

Ultimately, the only thing that really helps you through transition is the fact that it usually doesn't last for long. Hang on in there and scream, swear, shout, or do whatever gets you through. Let go, literally, and let your body take over: it's going to any minute now, anyway.

SEE IT THROUGH

Visualization techniques can help you get through tough times such as transition. For instance, imagine your pain is a crumbling brick that stands between you and your baby. Each contraction is like a wrecker's ball, smashing its way through and clearing your path. Focusing on a positive image, and the fact that you'll soon be holding your baby, will help you to stay in control and minimize the release of adrenaline, which can increase your perception of pain.

❊ During transition, a partner's place is in the wrong.

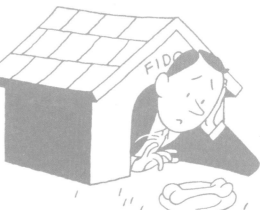

Coming ready or not

In the middle of the madness that is transition, someone will stick their fingers up your crotch to see if you've made it to 10 cm yet. Sorry, but this really is necessary. Your nurse-midwife has to make sure that the cervix is fully dilated before pushing so that the anterior lip—the front part of the cervix—doesn't tear. It's really important that you don't start pushing before this happens, because if this lip hasn't completely disappeared up into the uterus, it won't take kindly to being headbutted by the baby, and will swell up, making it even harder to get the baby out. So, don't push until you get the green light. Sounds easy, doesn't it? It is easy, until you get the urge to push. This urge is like opening the floodgates on the Hoover dam: the power behind it can be truly awesome. You're most likely to want to jump the gun if you're a mom who's already been through it all before, if you've got a butt full of poop, or if your baby is facing forward. If you've gone into premature labor, you may also get the urge to push before your cervix is fully dilated, but this isn't always a problem because your baby's head will be a little smaller than a full-termer.

So what can you do if your nurse-midwife says it's not time to push? Get down on all fours and shove your butt in the air. Yes, again. This takes the sting out of contractions, and may give the cervix a bit more space to do its thing. Moaning or wailing can channel some of the force out through your mouth, rather than down through your pelvis. It also helps to take short panting breaths in and out, or to puff out your cheeks (the ones on your face, that is) and blow out little spurts of air, as if you're blowing out a candle a few feet in front of you. Before doing any of these breathing tricks, make sure that your birth partner has a paper bag handy: one of those paper sickbags will do. Some women start to hyperventilate and get dizzy. If this happens, just breathe in and out of the bag for a moment or two until your head clears.

* Don't worry, ladies, I always warm my fingers up before I get to work!

Shape up

From here on, the shape of your pelvis, and the position that bumpsie has assumed, can have big impacts on your comfort zone and whether your delivery comes express or snail mail. Let's start with your bump. There are three basic positions it could assume: OAP and OPP, which are both headfirst, and the buttfirst breech position. OAP doesn't mean you're about to give birth to an old age pensioner, although some kids do come out looking like wrinkly old men. It stands for occipito anterior presentation, which is just a fancy way of saying that the baby is looking toward your spine and the back of its head, aka its occiput, is near the front of your belly. OPP, occipito posterior presentation, means that the back of the baby's head is against your spine, and it's looking out toward your belly. Some people say this position increases back labor, and it does tend to be a bit more uncomfortable. It also makes you want to push too soon.

You can spot the difference between OAP and OPP at a glance. OAP bumps are evenly rounded and almost semicircular in shape, while OPPs are top heavy and look a bit like an upside-down pear. The position of your placenta may determine whether bumpsie's an OAP or an OPP, because there is evidence that babies in the womb like to face their placenta, presumably to keep an eye on the pantry and oxygen supply.

Breech presentations are nowhere near as common as suggested by the movies. They happen in only 5 percent of deliveries at term, while the classic headfirst positions account for nearly 94.5 percent of deliveries. The other fraction of a percent is made up of some uncomfortable variations on the theme, like feet first, shoulder first, and even face first. Most of these babies can be delivered vaginally, but C-sections are becoming more widely used and a lot of these skills are being lost. Your chances of a vaginal delivery may depend on the age and experience of your nurse-midwife.

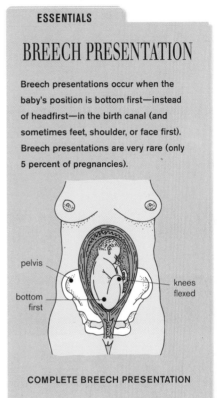

ESSENTIALS

BREECH PRESENTATION

Breech presentations occur when the baby's position is bottom first—instead of headfirst—in the birth canal (and sometimes feet, shoulder, or face first). Breech presentations are very rare (only 5 percent of pregnancies).

pelvis

knees flexed

bottom first

COMPLETE BREECH PRESENTATION

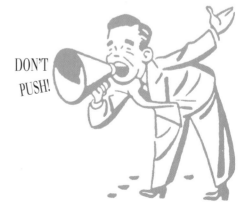

DON'T PUSH!

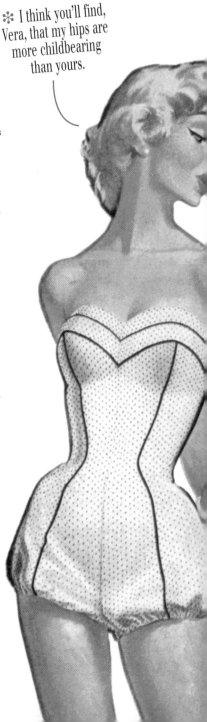

❊ I think you'll find, Vera, that my hips are more childbearing than yours.

Pelvis power

We bet you thought that all those cracks about childbearing hips were just catty lines dreamt up by gay men and thin women. Well, think again. There are actually four pelvic shapes, and the Rolls Royce when it comes to labor is known as the "gynecoid" pelvis. It's custom-built for the job. If you're of average build and height, and wear a size four shoe or bigger, you've probably got one: 50 percent of women have. The next best models are the anthropoid, displayed by 25 percent of women, and platypelloid, displayed by 5 percent. Women who are tall and have slim shoulders tend to be anthropoid, while platypelloids have a slightly flatter pelvis. Anthropoids are more likely to have an OPP baby and get back labor, while platypelloids sometimes hit a snag negotiating turns, but most come through without any major problems. The short straw goes to the androids, in more ways than one. One in five women has an android pelvis. As one textbook puts it, this pelvic shape is most likely to occur in "short and heavily built women who have a tendency to be hirsute." As if it's not bad enough being short, overweight, and hairy, these poor moms have deep pelvises that get narrower at the bottom, with angles that encourage baby to get stuck along the way.

Turning the other cheek

The second stage of delivery can take anything from a couple of minutes to three hours, but the average is around 30 minutes. It often brings a fresh surge of energy and an incredible sense of excitement, because the end—and pretty soon your baby's head—is in sight. As we've already mentioned, you'll get an incredible urge to push at some point around this time. It can come before you're fully dilated, as soon as you are, or sometimes not until the baby has slipped down a little more and is starting to press against your butt passage. By this time, the contractions are almost as regular as clockwork. They last longer, from 60 to 90 seconds, but you often get a longer rest in

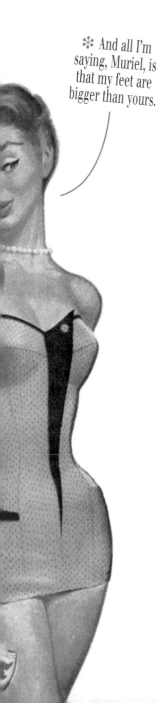

✳ And all I'm saying, Muriel, is that my feet are bigger than yours.

between, for around two to five minutes. They also feel very different. Early contractions are quite internalized and seem to encircle your belly, while the contractions in this second phase are much more expulsive, as if all force is coming down from your diaphragm and belly, and out through your legs.

When labor starts, the bit that is coming out first is known as the presenting part, although it bears only a passing resemblance to David Letterman. In the vast majority of cases, the presenting part is the baby's head, and at the start of the action your baby is most likely to be facing your back. This is also the most comfortable position for you. During the delivery, the baby will turn and twist to squeeze through your pelvis and sneak out under your pubic bone. This explains why some babies come out with pointy heads and faces like squashed frogs. Don't worry too much about squishing your baby. It's actually good for them to go through the wringer, because it gets their lungs ready for the outside world and squeezes out some of the amniotic fluid that's sloshing around in there. In the meantime, they're still getting plenty of oxygen pumped down the cord, and the skull is designed so that the bones can mold to your pelvis without damage.

Antenatal classes often illustrate this contortionist act with a dolly and a dismembered plastic pelvis. Unless you're planning to give birth to a Cabbage Patch doll, and don't mind losing your legs in the process, this is about as useful as showing you a needle and thread and explaining that the thread goes through the little hole in the needle. Most moms can figure out which bit goes where. What they want to know is how to get it there. The answers are: pushing, squeezing, and gravity. Finding the combination that works best for you is largely a matter of suck it and see. If you're feeling uncomfortable or progress is slowing, try another position and give it a couple of contractions before deciding if it's an improvement or not. There's also increasing evidence that gravity is a huge factor—well, it makes sense doesn't it?—so don't let anyone tell you to lie down unless you want to.

PUSHING THE RIGHT BUTTONS

There are two schools of thought when it comes to pushing during labor. The first is: relax, go slow, and gently does it; and the second is: go for it, girl! The more relaxed approach takes longer, but some women find it less stressful, and there's less chance of taking the spring out of your pelvic floor. The vigorous approach gets the job done quickly, and often comes naturally. To find out which method works best for you, listen to your body and go with the flow.

❖ Here come the cavalry, ma'am—we'll be right behind you.

However, you should listen to your nurse-midwife or physician too, because sometimes you might be desperate to push when it's actually better to hold back. If you're one of the few women who doesn't get the urge to push at all or you are too anesthetized, your nurse-midwife or physician will tell you when to bear down.

Some pregnancy books go on and on about remembering everything from your antenatal classes, and sticking to the breathing patterns and routines you've learned. Some even suggest that your birth partner should bring the book along to remind you of any advice you've forgotten. This, quite frankly, is nuts. If anyone had started quoting chapter and verse at me, I'd have thrown the book at them, literally. Try out the techniques you've been taught, but don't be afraid to discard any advice that isn't working. You won't be the first to find that theory is from Mars and practice is from Venus.

Whatever happens, you won't want to be lying down. If you're sitting or squatting, gravity will help to ease the baby down and out. You may get cramp in your legs, no matter how many practice squats you've done. Take a few breaths as the contraction builds, and then release them as you bear down, applying short spurts of pressure rather than one long push. In between contractions, take deep, regular breaths and relax as much as possible. Make a conscious effort to release any tension around your thighs and crotch. Focus on the rhythm of your contractions, so that any pressure you apply makes the most impact.

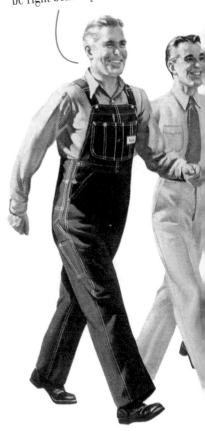

Some birth coaches, doulas, and antenatal teachers say you should never hold your breath and push, and they terrify women into compliance with dire tales about what could go wrong if you do. You could starve yourself and the baby of oxygen; you could burst so many blood vessels that you detach a retina or make your eyes bloodshot; you could shit yourself (big deal!); you could get so tense that your vagina seizes up. OK, hands up: I (and all the other moms I know) fell for this one. Like perfect little pupils, we channeled our energy into making lots of breathy moaning noises during each contraction, and managed to resist the urge to take a big, deep breath and PUSH! We panted and puffed, and wiggled our jaw to prevent tension. (Supposedly, if your jaw's not clenched, no other part of your body will be. Just for the record, this isn't true either.) There was only one snag with this passive approach: it's called a pelvis, and nothing is going to get through it without a bit of a shove. With each contraction, the head would appear in the doorway; but with each lull, it would slip back inside. This ludicrous game of peekaboo went on for almost an hour, with no sign of any real progress. Finally, we dumped the theory and did what came naturally, which was to hold a breath and push like mad. A matter of minutes later, the baby's head was crowning and it really was time to stop pushing.

We're not saying that pushing works for every woman or at every point, but if, like us, you're stuck in the middle of nowhere, it's worth trying. Forget the horror stories about lack of oxygen. They are, if you'll excuse the pun, rather overblown. Think about it: if we need air, reflex actions kick in, and we gasp for the stuff. It's no different when you're in labor. If you've ever had bad constipation, and most of us have at some point, you've probably already burst a blood vessel or two and survived the experience.

Once the baby's head starts to come into sight, you might be offered a mirror so that you can see what's going on. This can be fabulous and fascinating, or too gruesome for words: it's a matter of personal preference.

✳ What d'ya want to do with all this hot water, lady?

✳ Pa! Pa! Have we brought enough cigars?

Your nurse-midwife or physician might also suggest that you touch the head to feel the baby coming. This last bit is often a matter of two steps forward and one step back, with the baby's head pushing forward during contractions and then slipping back a fraction in between. Sometimes it's two steps forward and two steps back, and they'll have to call in the cavalry in the form of forceps or a vacuum extractor. Forceps look like oversize salad tongs, and fit around the baby's head. A vacuum extractor is a glorified vacuum cleaner, with a padded circular bit that fits onto the baby's head so that it can be sucked out. Both can cause a bit of misshaping and minor bruising. Any horror stories you've heard probably relate to "high forceps" procedures, which is another way of saying that they had to be put in a long way.

Sooner or later, the head stops slipping back. This is called crowning, but it's got nothing to do with glory, and it stings like hell. At this point, your nurse-midwife might guide your baby's head to stop it pushing forward too quickly and tearing your perineum (the skin and muscle between your vagina and butt). Throughout the second stage, it's gently stretched and opened out by the pressure of the baby's head (or butt, if it's a breech delivery), and this knocks out a lot, though not all, of the nerve endings. It also reduces blood loss from any tears or cuts. Once the head crowns, you have to stop pushing until your nurse-midwife gives the green light. This will give her time to check where the umbilical cord is—hopefully, it's not around your baby's neck—and a chance to ease your labia away from the baby's head. Take short panting breaths to stop yourself from pushing too soon. Some midwives massage the perineum as the baby's head crowns. This doesn't hurt, but there's no real evidence that it reduces tearing.

ESSENTIALS

FORCEPS

Forceps can be used to help guide the baby's head out of the birth canal. They should gently grip the sides of the baby's head, somewhere near the ears. If they have left marks anywhere else, it suggests someone got it wrong.

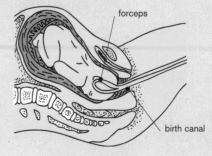

forceps

birth canal

FORCEPS DELIVERY

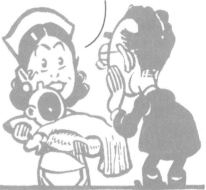

No, Mr. Brubaker, I'm afraid there isn't an off switch.

Sometimes the baby comes out quickly, with the head and shoulders both plopping out in one contraction. More commonly, it will take one contraction to push the head out, and a second to push the shoulders through. Once they're out, the rest of the baby slithers out. Dads who are watching should be warned that babies aren't squeaky clean and pink when they come out. They're covered with greasy white stuff called vernix and various bits of blood and gore, and some dads immediately panic and think that the baby is dead.

Forget all that stuff about holding the baby upside down and giving it a smack. Most start screaming before anyone's laid a finger on them, and if there is a problem, it's usually solved by suctioning any muck and fluid out of the mouth and windpipe. The cord is clamped and cut, and if you're breast-feeding you'll be encouraged to offer a booby as quickly as possible. This will release hormones that speed up the third stage. Immediately after the birth, you may feel drowsy, incredibly alert, elated, stunned, or almost anything else. You may also start to shiver uncontrollably.

The third stage is pushing out the placenta, which is a piece of cake after pushing out a baby. Actually, it's more like a piece of liver. Believe it or not, some women actually eat it. Personally, we'd rather stick matchsticks under our fingernails and listen to Barry Manilow's Greatest Hits 24 hours a day. For a fee, some companies freeze cord blood as an insurance policy against future health problems. Opinion on this one is divided, but it's definitely more effective than storing the placenta in your home freezer, as one mom we know has done for five years and counting. You may be given a shot of oxytocin to speed things up, and your nurse-midwife will check the placenta to make sure that there are no bits missing. Leftovers in the womb can cause hemorrhaging.

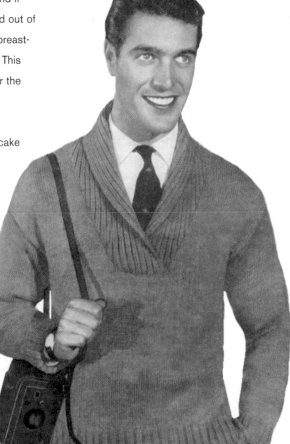

✻ Jeffrey was unnervingly pleased with his action shots of the third stage.

CUTTING TOO QUICK

If you have to have a forceps delivery or a vacuum delivery, or it looks as if you're going to tear really badly as the baby's head comes out, your nurse-midwife or physician may decide to cut the perineum. This, as all moms-in-the-making are well aware, is known as an episiotomy, and it's sometimes called the unkindest cut of all. Most moms, quite rightly, don't want an episiotomy, but doctors can't seem to agree on whether or not they are a good idea.

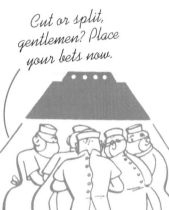

Cut or split, gentlemen? Place your bets now.

Unfortunately, it's the doctors who are the ones holding the scissors at the critical moment—if you're delivered by a physician, you're much more likely to be cut than if you're delivered by a nurse-midwife. Episiotomy rates vary hugely between different birth centers and individual carers, and even more between different parts of the world. In the United States, the national average is now down to 54 percent, although among private physicians it's still far too high at 65 percent. By contrast, one British study reported an episiotomy rate of just 10 percent when a "restrictive" policy—that is, cutting only when necessary, not "just in case"—was practiced.

The case for episiotomy is set out as follows: a controlled cut means that there's a smaller chance of a really bad tear, or of your pelvic floor muscles being so badly damaged that bits inside start slipping down, which is called a prolapse. Snippers also argue that an episiotomy is much easier to stitch up than a tear, and there's less risk of infection. The case against is that they're often unnecessary, always painful, and aren't actually any easier to repair. There's also no guarantee that a cut won't prevent further tearing, anyway. There's conflicting evidence on whether or not they help prevent long-term damage, and at least one study found that they actually do more harm than good. On balance, we think that in most cases you're better off saying, "Thanks, but no thanks," and taking your chances. In some situations, such as forceps or vacuum delivery, you may not have a choice. It makes sense to have an episiotomy if the baby's in

AFTERCARE

If you have stitches following an episiotomy or tear, it's important to change your sanitary pad frequently to minimize infection. Avoid touching the stitches and splash clean warm water over the area every time you've had a pee. Use gauze pads or a tissue to pat it dry, and take care to work from the front to the back.

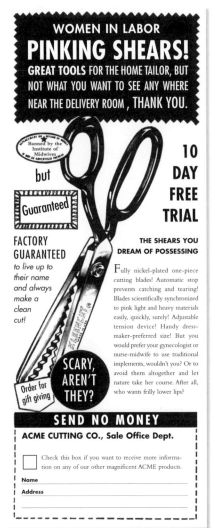

WOMEN IN LABOR

PINKING SHEARS!

GREAT TOOLS FOR THE HOME TAILOR, BUT NOT WHAT YOU WANT TO SEE ANY WHERE NEAR THE DELIVERY ROOM , THANK YOU.

Banned by the Institute of Midwives

but

Guaranteed

10 DAY FREE TRIAL

FACTORY GUARANTEED

to live up to their name and always make a clean cut!

THE SHEARS YOU DREAM OF POSSESSING

Fully nickel-plated one-piece cutting blades! Automatic stop prevents catching and tearing! Blades scientifically synchronized to pink light and heavy materials easily, quickly, surely! Adjustable tension device! Handy dress-maker-preferred size! But you would prefer your gynecologist or nurse-midwife to use traditional implements, wouldn't you? Or to avoid them altogether and let nature take her course. After all, who wants frilly lower lips?

SCARY, AREN'T THEY?

Order for gift giving

SEND NO MONEY

ACME CUTTING CO., Sale Office Dept.

☐ Check this box if you want to receive more information on any of our other magnificent ACME products.

Name

Address

distress and must be delivered quickly; if your nurse-midwife or physician has to make room for forceps or a vacuum extractor in the event of an assisted delivery; and if there's a risk of brain damage due to the baby's head being squashed in a preterm or breech delivery. It doesn't make sense to do one "just in case," to hurry things along when mom and baby are fine, or because that's the way your birth center or physician handles each delivery.

If you've got to have an episiotomy, you'll be given a shot of lidocaine to deaden the area. Your carer will put two fingers inside your vagina to position the scissors and then make a single cut, about 4 cm long, during a contraction. In the United States, this is usually a median cut, which is a straight line down from the vagina toward your butt. In the UK, it's more likely to be a mediolateral cut, which is at about seven o'clock. A median cut reduces blood loss, is easier to repair, and doesn't hurt so much, but it is also more likely to damage your sphincter, the muscle that keeps your butt shut.

Tearaways

If you do tear during delivery, the damage is often superficial. If it's in the top bit of your labia, it may not need stitching at all, depending on how much it's bleeding. Tears heading the other way, toward your butt, are classified by degrees. A first degree tear involves the labial bits that are usually moist; a second degree tear goes past them and into a tiny bit of perineal muscle; a third degree tear involves damage to the sphincter muscle; a fourth degree tear goes all the way down to your back passage. First and second degree tears are no big deal and are easily patched up, but you'll need more local anesthetic for third and fourth degree ones. If any needlework is required, it's done as quickly as possible to reduce blood loss and pain.

CESARS—IT'S NOT CUT-AND-DRIED

There's a myth that C-sections are named after Julius Caesar, who was supposedly delivered surgically. Actually, it comes from the Roman law known as Lex Caesare, which said that if a woman died in advanced pregnancy the baby should be cut out and buried separately. Some such babies had other ideas and started screaming. There's an even crazier myth that they're a shortcut to painfree, no fuss deliveries. They ain't!

C-section rates vary dramatically. Brazilian women love them: 90 percent of moms in Rio go for the cut, and one celebrity even scheduled her delivery so that it could be shown on primetime TV. We'd rather watch nail polish dry. In the United States, C-section rates peaked at around 40 percent in the 1980s, but now run at around 25 percent, although some private physicians do two or three times as many. In the UK, the number has been climbing steadily, from around 10 percent in the 1980s to just over 20 percent now.

There are lots of reasons for the increase. Doctors are so scared of getting sued that they don't want to take any chances. Some women, like the babes from Brazil, labor (mentally, that is) under the mistaken belief that a vaginal delivery will screw up their sex lives. Others just don't like the thought of pain during the delivery. They forget that they're just postponing the inevitable, and will have even more pain when they've got the baby to deal with, too.

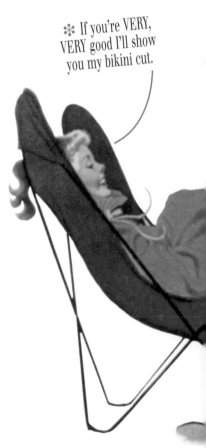

❋ If you're VERY, VERY good I'll show you my bikini cut.

Why have one?

Good reasons for having an elective C-section include: breech presentation; a low-lying placenta (placenta previa); a tiny pelvis and a big baby; really bad rhesus incompatibility; in some cases of twins and active genital herpes. Gray areas include previous surgery or C-sections and not such good reasons include: a fear of pain (you'll get it anyway); convenience (whose?); worries that your love canal will turn into the Grand

PRIME CUTS

The skin incision, known as pfanensteel, is a 4-inch (10-cm) horizontal cut along the bikini line. A vertical skin incision would only be carried out in life-threatening emergencies. There are two types of uterine incision: the low flap transverse and, in rare cases, a classical vertical incision.

Canal (that's what Kegels are for); or because Madonna had one (she also posed for a soft-porn coffee table book, and it's our guess you won't be copying her on that). Of course, it's a woman's right to choose, so long as it's an informed choice.

Emergency Cesarians are necessitated by a different kettle of complications, such as pre-eclampsia, fetal distress, obstruction, cord prolapse, and detached placenta. By far the most common reason for having a C-section is that you've had one before—which is a pretty good reason for avoiding one in the first place. However, a vaginal birth after Cesarean (VBAC) can be attempted with good success if a lower uterine incision was made at the time of the previous C-section (a horizontal cut called a low flap transverse).

If you're having one, the pain relief will vary (an elective C-section leaves time for an epidural or spinal block and you'll be awake during the delivery, while an emergency C-section can occasionally necessitate a general anesthetic when time is of the essence), but the procedure's the same.

What happens

The top bit of your pubic hair will be shaved and you may be fitted into anti-embolism stockings, which make budget-buy pantihose look like pure silk luxury. You'll have an IV drip put into your arm, and then either an epidural or general anesthetic, depending on the urgency. Once the pain relief kicks in, a little tube called a catheter is stuck up your urethra so that you can pee into a bag, and your tummy will be basted with antiseptic ready for the cut. It takes only about five minutes to get the baby and placenta out, and another 35 or 40 minutes to suck out all the amniotic fluid (don't be surprised if you hear all sorts of strange gurgling sounds), and stitch and staple everything up again. You'll be given a shot of oxytocin to prevent bleeding, and more pain relief.

Yowl
Yowl
Yowl

Aftershock
IT'S ONLY JUST BEGUN

Phew, you're thinking, I'm glad that's all over. Think again, honey. As you look at your little bundle of joy—or puking and screaming little bundle, as the case may be—you may find yourself wondering how something so small can have been responsible for so much upheaval. As Karen Carpenter used to sing, "We've only just begun"—you're now a Parent, with a capital P...

Immediately after the birth, your baby performs a bit of do-it-yourself heart surgery. While he or she was inside you, both sides of the baby's heart beat at the same time, and oxygenated blood from the cord pumped into both sides. Your baby's first breath alters the pressure in the lungs, and closes down the arteries that used to bring blood from the cord. This, in turn, shuts down ducts in the heart, so that the two sides start working independently—one taking delivery of oxygenated blood from the lungs and dispatching it around the body, the other taking delivery of the used blood from the body and sending it back to the lungs. Clever little things, aren't they?

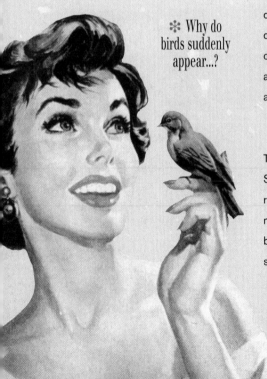

❋ Why do
birds suddenly
appear...?

Apgar and knowing the score

This is when your baby sits his or her first test, resulting in an Apgar score. Some people say this stands for appearance, pulse, grimace, activity, and respiration, and those are basically the things that it rates. It's actually named after the anesthetist, Virginia Apgar, who came up with it (if it had been devised by Vernon Apgar, I probably wouldn't have to point this out), so let's give credit where it's due. The test gives a score of zero, one, or two points to five characteristics: color, heartbeat, response to stimulus, muscle tone, and breathing. The lowest score would go to a blue, limp baby who has no heartbeat, doesn't move, and makes no attempt to breathe.

(Most of us would call this "dead.") A perfect ten would go to a crying, squirming, pink baby who coughs or sneezes, and has a heart rate of more than 100 bpm. Anything above seven means the baby's in good shape; anything below means it needs extra help. Your nurse-midwife or physician will suggest a shot, or oral drops, of vitamin K to prevent hemorrhaging (although babies do start making their own, using gut bacteria, after 48 hours). In many hospitals, eye drops such as erythromycin and penicillin, may be given.

While all this is going on, your baby will also be weighed and measured. These figures generate more interest than a diet club weigh-in. At the top of the FAQ list over the next few days will be queries about your baby's gender, weight, and how long it took to get it out. The average newborn weighs 7½ pounds (3.4 kg), but boys tend to be a bit heavier, and the babies of smokers usually weigh less. Anything from 5 pounds, 10 ounces (2.6 kg) to 9 pounds (4.08 kg) is considered normal for a baby who's gone the full distance. Don't panic if your baby's already showing nonconformist tendencies: he or she can still be perfectly healthy outside these guidelines.

Most babies are around 21 inches (53 cm) long when they come out, but normal proportions can range from the equivalent of a Tom Cruise to the equivalent of a Michael Jordan. It's the head measurement that your physician will be most interested in. The average is about 14 inches (35.5 cm) around, and any extreme (and we do mean extreme) variations can be signs of trouble. The tale of the tape is often delayed for a day or two, because labor squashes the baby's head out of shape.

Other tests and checks include jiggling the baby's legs around to make sure that they fit into their hip sockets properly—this is easily corrected, but the sooner it's sorted out the better—and looking your gift horse in the mouth to make sure that everything's joined up properly. There's also, of course, a quick count of body parts to make sure nothing's missing.

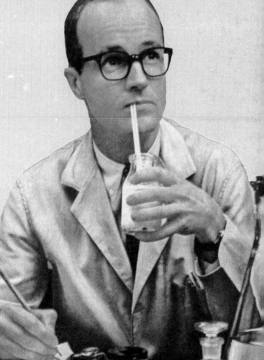

❊ Norbert finally passed the Apgar test after his fourth resit.

There are a few kneejerk reactions to try out—the baby's, that is, not yours. One involves standing your baby upright to see if he or she will try to walk. If he or she does, it doesn't mean that you've produced a prodigy, or that it's time to send out for baby's first Blahniks: all babies should do this at first, it's a primitive reflex that disappears sometime around three months. A finger will be placed against the baby's palm to see whether his or her hand will slam shut and grab the finger tighter than a drowning man can grab a rope: this tests the grasp reflex, obviously enough.

FROG OR BABY?

Surprise appearance

In the movies, newborn babies are deliciously plump and pink, and gaze up at their moms with adoration. That's because welfare laws ban newborns from movie sets. Newborn babies are actually more likely to resemble squashed frogs, Winston Churchill, pointy-headed aliens, or morphs of all three. A newborn will also have a stump of umbilical cord, secured with a plastic clip that looks like one of those store security tags that sets off the door alarm when the shop assistant forgets to take it off. The stump itself will look more and more like ET's finger until it finally drops off. Other delicious traits of newborns include: puffy, bruised eyes; zits (they're called milia, and are caused by a temporary blockage of sebaceous glands); tits and swollen genitals (from mom's hormones); fine hair all over the body (it's called lanugo, and usually rubs off in a week or two); "Mongolian spots" (blue-gray blotches on the back and butt, common among Asian and dark skinned babies); and "stork marks," red marks at the back of the neck where Old Mister Stork was holding the baby in his beak. (You mean you didn't see him fly by with that flock of pigs?)

BOUNCING BABIES

One reflex test your physician will try is to lift the baby slightly, and let him or her fall down onto the physician's hand. The baby should be startled into a Moro reflex—who wouldn't be if some strange giant threatened to drop them? The Moro reflex is a fancy way of saying that the baby tries to break the fall by throwing out the arms and legs.

It's all in the wrist!

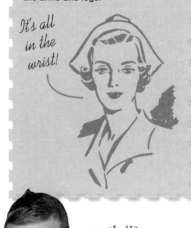

✳ Who you callin' a squashed frog?

If your baby was being monitored more closely than a moon shot during his or her descent, there may be a little red scratch on the top of the head where the sensor was clipped on while it was still on the way out. It's quite easy to attach one once the cervix is dilated or the baby's already in the birth canal. This disappears in a day or two. The head itself can also be pointy, or flattened on the sides, from being squashed through the vagina or gripped by forceps. There might be a round, raised bit where a vacuum extractor was stuck on. These things disappear in a day or two. There's also a soft spot toward the front of the head, called the fontanelle, where you may be able to see a vein pulse with each heartbeat. What you don't want to see is deflation or sinking here, because these are signs of dehydration.

Other things that your mom may not have told you about include periods and poop. Baby girls sometimes get a tiny bit of bleeding from the vagina, and if nobody's warned you about it this can be a real shocker. It happens because there's been so much estrogen sloshing around your body that some of it has spilled over the placenta and into your baby. It's perfectly harmless, and soon disappears.

Then there's our old friend, meconium. If, like me, there were times when it felt as though your body had been taken over by an alien, your first close encounter of the meconium kind will have you on the phone to Mulder and Scully warning them to open another X-File. Meconium doesn't smell, but it looks foul—like greenish-black sticky tar—and for the first two or three days that's all that comes out of your baby's butt. By about day three all this accumulated crap will have been expelled, and your baby will start doing proper poops—well, proper poops for a baby. Breast-fed babies produce sloppy yellow stuff that looks like grain mustard, while bottle-fed babies make harder poops, and sometimes have a tough time getting them out. However they're being fed, babies often get a blister in the middle of the upper lip from all that sucking.

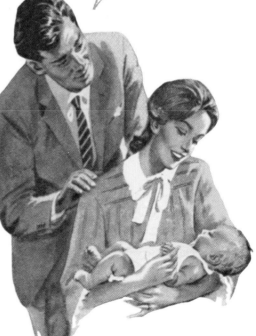

She's lovely, darling, but any more meconium leakage and she goes straight back to the factory.

SQUASHED FROGS AND ALIENS BABY E.T.s

I f you prepare yourself for a hairy, squashed frog with zits and you actually get a cherub, you'll be doubly delighted. Whatever your baby looks like, he or she is your cherub, or squashed frog, and you may fall in love at first sight. Or you may not. It's not compulsory, and not everyone does. Some women are so exhausted that they're numb to the whole experience, while others are so energized that they can't sleep for hours, even though they're exhausted.

✳ And that demented toothy alien in the fishtank is your father, young man.

Seeing your baby for the first time can be magical, overwhelming, awe-inspiring, or terrifying. Whatever you're feeling, it's OK. This is the real world, not a mushy romantic novel, and rose-tinted glasses aren't standard issue in hospital labor wards. Whatever you're feeling, you certainly won't be the first to feel it. There's a whole rollercoaster of emotions to come, so this particular one won't last for long.

Your delivery will also have a huge impact on your first reactions. If it was a relatively quick and easy labor, you're much more likely to be upbeat. If you've been pushing for hours, and feel bruised, battered, and shattered, you might find it hard not to associate your baby with your aching butt.

We're not saints, and it's not a sin, so don't beat yourself up if you don't bond like glue. There's plenty of time yet.

Green-eyed monsters

New moms sometimes find it hard to talk about these reactions, but other members of the family might not hold back, particularly older brothers or sisters. They don't call it sibling rivalry for nothing, and if you're not careful, this is where it starts. Kids, particularly toddlers, can come out with the most amazing lines: "OK, we've seen the baby, can we send it back now?"; "But it's a boy, I wanted a girl!"; "I don't like this one, can we have a different one?"; "What's wrong with her, why can't she play football?"

Head off antagonism with a bribe. Give the older children a present from the baby to make them feel that it's a special day for them, too. Ask visitors not to bring presents for the baby unless they also bring something for older children. Don't be too offended if they do decide to come empty handed: it's infinitely better than enduring a toddler's hissy fit.

It's also important to ask visitors to make as much fuss—or perhaps even more fuss—of other children as they do of the new baby. Friends and family with young children of their own are generally pretty good on this one—they may have been there, not done it this way, and still have the bruised shins to prove it. Parents and grandparents are more likely to need a little extra coaching. If you've got one of those utterly impossible older relations who thinks this is all a lot of mollycoddling new age nonsense, and refuses to toe the line, don't even think about arguing: there's just no point. Simply tell them, in the nicest possible way of course, that they either do it your way, or they don't do it at all. Period. If necessary, blame it on your hormones, but do it. Even with moms, you may ask? Especially with moms! If you don't get the ground rules right from the very beginning—and make sure that they're your ground rules, not your mom's, mom-in-law's, or anyone else's—you may soon be wishing that the ground would open up and swallow you, or them.

You see before you the helpless victim of a savage, all-out knitting war between rival granny gangs.

While we're on the subject of visitors, you don't have to see them if you're feeling too tired, too crummy, or just don't want to deal with someone right away. Make it clear to friends and family that they should check with your partner before popping in. If necessary, fib and say that the hospital's very strict about the number of visitors you're allowed. Your partner could stick around during visiting times and maneuver people toward the exit if they're staying too long—some people just don't seem to know when to leave.

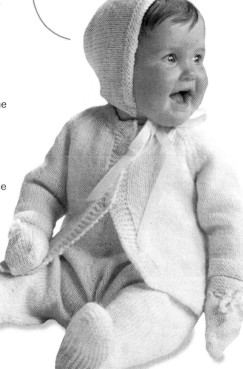

THE AFTERMATH SORE POINTS

Immediately after the birth, you may feel lousy or you may feel euphoric and upbeat until the sleepless nights kick in. Your crotch will probably be swollen and sore; you'll be bleeding what seems like bucketloads; your tits will ache; your bump will have collapsed into a pile of blubber that wobbles like a jelly on a plate; you will feel as though you're still having contractions; having a pee will probably be excruciating; and you'll be frightened to have a poop in case something crucial falls out.

You might also have bloodshot eyes and bruising on your cheeks (both sets) from all that pushing; you might find it hard to take deep breaths because your ribs ache so much, for the same reason; you may be drowning in sweat, due to a combination of hormones and overheating in hospitals; and you'll still be walking like John Wayne, for obvious reasons. If you've had a C-section, you won't have crotch pain—instead, you'll feel as if you've been kicked in the guts by a team of mules—but, other than that, the picture will be much the same.

Your pussy will probably feel bruised, swollen, and very sore—in short, it will feel as if it's been in a fight with a pack of Rottweilers. This feeling won't last long. Ask your partner to buy some rubber gloves, fill them up with water, tie the ends tightly, and then put them in the freezer. When they're half-frozen, you can mold them into icy hands that will reach all the bits that the other remedies can't. (Palmside up with the middle finger sticking up at a right angle is good.) Alternatively, ask your physician or nurse-midwife for some rubber surgical gloves and fill them with crushed ice. Sitting on a bag of frozen peas works, too. Forget all those stories about using rubber rings, they only focus pressure on your pussy and make it hurt even more.

❊ Did you know that the Duke took lessons from new moms to get his moseyin' stroll just right?

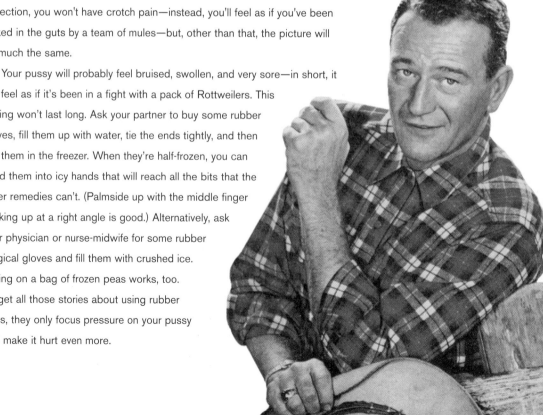

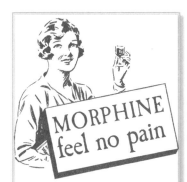

When your elders give you a hard time about your birthing skills, remember that this is what they had to help them, while you are getting by on a cup of camomile and aromatherapy.

The supreme tonic restorative

In Anemia, Depression, Debility, Sleeplessness, and Nervous troubles, never fails to bring back health and strength.

Available in LARGE MEDIUM SMALL   *Available from Wine Merchants and Grocers*

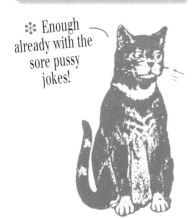

❋ Enough already with the sore pussy jokes!

C you later

AFTER C-SECTION

You won't need the helping hands and frozen peas if you've had a C-section, but you will definitely need some heavy-duty pain relief, such as morphine or synthetic narcotics such as Percocet. Your initial recovery will depend a great deal on whether you've had a general anesthetic, spinal block, or epidural, and how your body has reacted. Some people find that they feel extremely woozy and nauseous after having had a general, while others can shake them off quite quickly. (Your capacity for alcohol and tendency to get hangovers is sometimes a clue to how you will react, because booze and anesthetics target similar parts of the brain.) Weird dreams and hallucinations are common, and you may feel as disoriented as an Englishman in New York. If you've had an epidural or spinal block, sensation will return from the toes up, and you'll be encouraged to wiggle them.

After a C-section, you'll have to pee through a catheter. This is usually removed on the first day after delivery. Some doctors still prefer it if you don't eat any food right after delivery (you'll probably be too exhausted to think about food anyway!). Many doctors, though, will now allow women to drink shortly afterward if they are not nauseous or vomiting and allow them to eat on the first day if they are hungry. Solid foods should be no problem once you are passing gas (that's when you've done your first butt burp to you and me) because it's a good sign that normal bowel function is recovering. As soon as you're wheeled out of the operating room, your baby should be tucked up into bed beside you. If the baby has to go into the SCBU or NICU for any reason, you'll be given a Polaroid to cuddle instead. It's a nice thought, but it ain't the same.

You'll be encouraged to try to get up as soon as possible, which can be anywhere between eight and 24 hours after surgery. A nurse will help you up, but you'll be moving very slowly—rather like a mummy in a B-grade

❋ You would never guess I was doing my Kegel exercises...my lips hardly move at all.

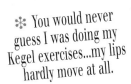

horror movie. You may feel dizzy, weak, and wobbly; you'll definitely feel excruciating pain. However, these small steps are giant leaps for womankind on the road to recovery. Resist the temptation to bend over like the Hunchback of Notre Dame (that's the cathedral in Paris, not the university). The sooner you can stand up straight and start moving (well, shuffling along), the quicker the pain goes away.

It will hurt not only when you laugh, but also when you cough, sneeze, or fart. These activities won't feel quite so bad if you bend your knees and hold a pillow against your stitches. The bowels are shut down for the duration of the surgery, so trapped gas can be a real problem afterward. Try lying on your side and breathing deeply, or making little coughing noises; this can help to release it.

Put the squeeze on

Kegels aren't quite so important when you've had a C-section, but they're crucial when you've given birth in the old-fashioned way. Start doing them as soon as possible, and as often as you can. It might hurt a bit at first, and your pussy will probably feel like a Mills and Boon heroine—all weak and trembly—but the more you do your pelvic floor exercises, the quicker everything gets back into shape. It also speeds up the healing process by stimulating circulation. Be warned: if you slack on your Kegels, everything down below will go slack, too. You'll probably end up peeing yourself when you laugh, cough, or sneeze, and incontinence is no joke. If you don't get your pelvic floor back into shape, it will get floppier and floppier as you get older and/or have more children. After menopause, your innards may even attempt to become your outards, and your womb will feel as if it's falling out of your ass. Has that frightened you? Good—now go and do your Kegels.

Mind your pees and poops

Your first pee and poop are like great leaps into the unknown, and you might have to screw up your courage to take your first tentative push. It will help if you eat plenty of fiber, and drink lots of water. Don't worry if it feels as though your pelvic floor muscles are about to go down the drain: nothing's going to fall out that isn't meant to. It helps to hold some toilet tissue against your perineum to give it a bit more support. Some women don't poop for a few days, or even a week, but that only clogs things up even more. It's a good idea to get off your butt: gentle exercise will help to get things moving along. Eat as much fruit as you can. If all else fails, take a mild laxative.

Your butt might have grown a frilly collar of hemorrhoids that were pushed out along with the baby—how attractive! Sometimes they go back inside of their own accord, but don't be embarrassed about mentioning them to your nurse-midwife or physician, particularly if they're painful or bleeding. Icepacks and hemorrhoid creams will help to relieve the pain. (Also, if the bags under your eyes are so bad that they're carrying Guccis of their own, dab a bit of hemorrhoid cream on them as well. Seriously, it really works. There isn't a supermodel worth her Chanel who leaves home without her butt cream.) Hospital toilet tissue can sometimes be as smooth as sandpaper, so ask your partner to bring along the softest, most luxurious brand he can buy.

Peeing can be painful if you have stitches or tears, or needed a catheter. When you take your first pee, try to lean forward as much as possible to steer the flow away from your perineum, or use a jug to pour cool water over your crotch as you're peeing. A lukewarm bath with five or six drops of tea tree oil is very soothing and mildly antiseptic. A little salt helps too, so long as you don't try rubbing it into the wounds. Gently wash your stitches at least twice a day. Don't get into a lather with soap—

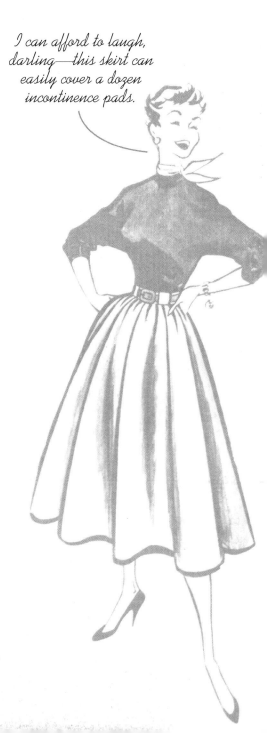

I can afford to laugh, darling—this skirt can easily cover a dozen incontinence pads.

ouch!—just splash on some cool water or dip your butt into a bath. Pat your pussy dry, or fan it dry with a newspaper or magazine. Blowdrying it with a hairdryer is definitely not a good idea.

Don't panic at the amount of blood you'll be losing. It's called lochia, and it's perfectly normal, even when it seems to gush like Old Faithful as you get out of bed. You'll leak lochia for two or three weeks. At first it will be bright red, then it turns a faded pink, then brown, and finally yellowish-white. Use highly absorbent sanitary pads, not tampons—apart from the ouch factor, they increase the risk of infection and probably won't cope with the flow anyway. One of the many benefits of breast-feeding is that it releases hormones which speed up the healing of the uterus by cranking up uterine contractions. The first time around, you might not even notice these contractions, but if you've already had a child they can be quite strong and painful. If they're really bad, take an acetaminophen-based painkiller.

Milk it, ladies!

The best remedy for sore or chapped nipples is simple and easily to hand—breast milk. After each feed, squirt a little breast milk out and rub it around the nipple and areola. Leave it to dry naturally, in the sunshine if you can. If you're in a hurry, you can just fan them dry with a newspaper.

Nipple problems in the bud

If you're breast-feeding, the first couple of days can be hell. The pain is supposed to peak around feed number 20, but personally I was too busy cursing to count. Until now, your nipples functioned as delicate little love buttons. After a day or two of being sucked incessantly, they'll have all the sensitivity of Barbara Walters interviewing Osama bin Laden. The nerve endings will finally shut down for the duration, and your nipples will develop the durability and texture of old rubber. However, before you get this hardened, it can be tough. Your nipples might become so sore and chapped that they start cracking up, taking you along with them. Avoid nipple creams and lotions, even the supposedly natural ones. Comfrey, for instance, which has been used in some herbal nipple creams, has been linked to liver damage,

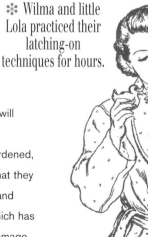

❄ Wilma and little Lola practiced their latching-on techniques for hours.

and in many parts of the world comfrey products are banned. Getting the baby to latch on properly (more on that later, *see pages 206–209*) will help to head off problems, and if you suddenly hit problems after a period of success, ask your physician to rule out thrush.

Around the third day, when colostrum gives way to proper milk, your tits will probably be huge, feel rock hard and red hot, and ache like hell. This is called engorgement, and the good news is that it doesn't last: it's just a hiccup while your body finds the right balance between supply and demand. You can minimize these problems by starting to breast-feed as soon as possible. Screw the hospital schedules if anyone says it's not convenient. If your boobies feel like balloons that are about to burst, squeeze off a little milk to relieve the pressure. Alternating hot and cold towels will also help, but the best soother of all is chilled cabbage leaves tucked into your bra. How on earth this was discovered is a mystery, but it really does work. Some women say that the crinkly savoy cabbages are the best, but any type is effective. The only downside is that the leaves almost start to cook, and fill the air with an unmistakable, and distinctly unappetizing, aroma.

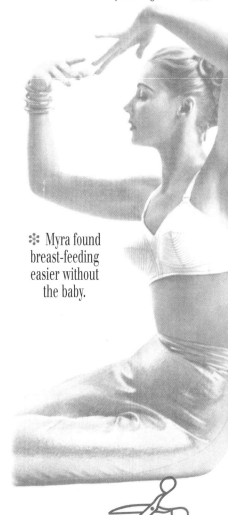

❊ Myra found breast-feeding easier without the baby.

Clip and Mail Today!

Savoy: the Facts
The Breast-Friendly Brassica
Verona Late

This Free Booklet

MAY BE WORTH YOUR SANITY

SAVOY CABBAGE HAS IT ALL! VITAMIN C, FIBER, FOLATE, AND BETA CAROTENE! PLUS EACH LEAF MAKES A COOLING, CALMING POULTICE FOR ENGORGED BREASTS!

Read about all these great benefits, and more, in our lavish, free booklet! Send no money but waste no time! Mail this form today, and we will rush you your very own copy instantly!

Name

Address

Phone

GOING WITH THE FLOW ALL ABOUT BREAST-FEEDING

Breast-feeding can be a touchy subject for some people, and we don't just mean for the dinosaurs who turn a deeper shade of purple than Barney when they see it being done in public. We've already covered a lot of the benefits of breast-feeding (*see pages 132–134*), but what about the practicalities? It's not actually that difficult: women have been doing it for centuries without needing to take a degree course in lactation and latching on. However, there's a hell of a lot of conflicting advice out there.

❊ Annabel despaired at the amount of theory that went into breast-feeding.

POOP FACT

Whatever goes in at one end, comes out the other—your new arrival will need around 50 clean diapers a week (you can rotate 20 cloth ones). This load will get lighter as Junior gets more efficient at dumping his or her load, if you get our drift.

Unfortunately some of this conflicting advice comes from people who should really know better, like (whisper it) nurse-midwives. We're talking about long lists of foods that you should eat, and even longer lists of foods that you shouldn't eat. Some nurse-midwives will grab your tit with one hand and your baby's head with the other, and shove them together as if they were slapping plaster on a wall. Ignore any advice from women who haven't themselves breast-fed for at least three months. If they wouldn't, or couldn't, get it right themselves, they're as much use to you as snowshoes in California.

Here are some other fascinating—well, we think so—facts about breast-feeding: your baby might headbutt your boobies to let you know that he or she is hungry (it's called rooting, and some people say it helps the let-down reflex that gets milk flowing); your boobies may hurt and squirt milk when your baby cries (it's a neat evolutionary trick to make sure that babies go to the top of your priorities when they need feeding); and babies can make the most extraordinary snorting noises when feeding, prompting you to check that it is a baby down there and not a piglet.

In France and some other countries, women are legally entitled to bare their breasts while feeding. We reckon that this makes a lot more sense than the right to bear arms. However, you don't have to be an exhibitionist to breast-feed in public: that's what pashminas are for. On one occasion I was traveling across London during the rush hour when my daughter decided

ESSENTIALS

HOME TRUTHS THAT AREN'T TRUE

Here are some of the breast-feeding fallacies that you might encounter

"Both breasts should be used at each feed."

☞ Why? It's not as if the unused milk is going to go bad, and the worst that can happen is that you might look a bit lopsided.

"You can't breast-feed if your baby is born prematurely."

☞ Piffle. Preterm babies have the most to gain from breast-feeding. Milk made by moms whose babies have arrived early is quite different from the milk made by moms whose babies arrived on schedule and the nutrient balance adjusts automatically to your baby's changing needs. Babies born more than six weeks early may not have a developed sucking reflex, but if your baby is being tube fed, it's better for them to have expressed breast milk than formula.

"Put a time limit on feeding during the first few days to prevent nipple soreness."

☞ This won't help your nipples, it will screw up your milk supply, and it will infuriate your baby.

"The baby should feed for ten minutes on each breast, and feeds should last no longer than 20 minutes."

☞ Let babies feed for as long as they want. There are times when it will feel as if that's all day long. Babies are just like us: sometimes they fancy a snack, sometimes they want a major pig-out.

"Give your baby a top-off with formula if they seem hungry."

☞ Absolutely not. Supplementing breast-feeds with formula screws up the delicate balance of supply and demand and you will end up with an even hungrier baby because you're making less milk.

"The baby should be fed at regular intervals, even if it means waking them up."

☞ Who dreamed this one up? Sleeping babies are like sleeping dogs: always let them lie. They'll let you know when they're hungry.

"You have to hold your breast away from the baby's nose."

☞ If it's in the way, your baby will simply stop sucking.

"Colostrum is too thin and watery to satisfy a baby."

☞ This is absolute nonsense: it might not look like much, but colostrum is packed with protein and immune-boosting antibodies.

✳ I like the furry one best—he's quiet and he never makes a mess.

✳ When's she gonna unbutton the gingham? I'm starving.

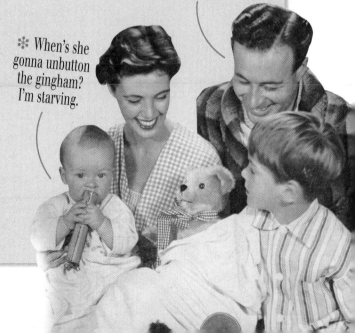

ESSENTIALS

HOME TRUTHS THAT HELP

Here are a few breast-feeding tips that really will help

☞ Make sure you're sitting comfortably and, if it helps, use a pillow to support your baby or your back. This is important if you're having attachment problems—the physical ones—or are feeding twins.

☞ Position the baby horizontally across your tummy, with the mouth directly over the target. Aim to get as much of the breast in as possible: not just the bull's-eye of the nipple, but some of the surrounding circle (the areola) as well. Some people say you should get all of the areola into the baby's mouth. This is fine if it's only 1–2 inches (2.5–5 cm) across, but if you've got areola the size of poached eggs—your baby won't have a chance to suck. The nipple should be near the top of your baby's mouth, and the lower lip should be as far away as possible.

☞ Have a snack and a drink within easy reach. These days, the advice is to stick to something non-alcoholic and decaffeinated, but back in the 1950s some books suggested something stronger, plus a cigarette, to help you relax. This proves how silly some advice can be! The point about relaxation is valid, though: the more you worry and tense up, the more likely you are to lose the flow.

☞ Feed on demand, and don't worry about running out. Breast-feeding is all about supply and demand: the more your baby demands, the more you'll be able to supply. Topping off with a bottle of baby formula will sabotage breast-feeding, because you'll just end up making less milk.

☞ Don't wash your breasts before feeding. There's absolutely no need, and there's some evidence that not washing them encourages the presence of friendly bacteria that help your baby to make its own supply of vitamin K.

☞ Some babies are a bit like some men: they like falling asleep with a nipple in their mouth. If you think your baby has stopped feeding, look for signs of movement around the cheek and jawline. If you think he or she might still be hungry, or you want him or her to get on with it, stroke his or her cheek with your finger. If your baby has fallen asleep at the breast, don't just pull him or her off: it's like sticking your nipple down a vacuum cleaner. Release the suction by wriggling your little finger into the mouth so that your nipple

is released with a painless pop. If breast-feeding hurts for any longer than a few seconds, take your baby off the nipple in this way and alter the position.

☞ Sometimes it may feel as if your nipples are being pierced by needles when the first squirts of milk come out. This will only last for a second or two, but it often helps to prime the pumps first by squeezing out a little bit of milk.

☞ After each feed, squeeze out a little milk, and leave it to dry on your nipples. It's more effective than commercial nipple creams, and it won't leave a nasty taste in your baby's mouth. Sunlight helps the nipples to heal, too. If your nipples are really badly chapped, try using nipple shields, or expressing milk and giving it back to your baby in a bottle.

that she had to be fed, NOW! I tucked her under a large wrap, unbuttoned a shirt button or two, and let her tuck in. By the time she had finished, there'd been an almost complete turnover of passengers and apart from another mom who was in on the secret and kept shooting me amused looks, none of the other passengers had a clue what I was up to. You could almost hear the clunk of jaws dropping when I'd buttoned up again and proceeded to slip a very content and sleepy baby out from under my wrap.

One strange thing about breast-feeding is that you can never predict who's going to throw a fit. Wentworth—one of England's most prestigious, and (you'd think) snootiest, golf clubs—didn't turn a well-groomed hair when I fed my daughter in a quiet corner of the clubroom, but mediocre restaurants with food that's more cordon blur than cordon bleu have blown gaskets. Quite frankly, if it really does upset someone that much, then it's their problem, not yours, and certainly not your baby's. Feign deafness, or a lack of English, or just plain ignore them.

Much the same advice goes for dealing with the busybodies who feel it's their duty to tell moms who bottle-feed how much damage they're doing to their babies. OK, breast is best, but baby formula is a lot better than it used to be, and it's miles better than cow's milk. (Although formula is made from cow's milk, it's specially adapted to make it more easily digestible, and is fortified with extra iron and some vitamins.) Heavens above, the way some of the anti-bottle brigade talk, you'd think moms were feeding their babies neat vodka. Millions of perfectly healthy adults were raised on infant formula. Buy an age-appropriate formula, follow the directions scrupulously, and always store made-up bottles in the main part of the refrigerator, because the temperature in door compartments isn't always cold enough.

※ Mmmmm I'd definitely say breast is best!

LADIES SING THE BLUES

The hormones that made your life hell during pregnancy don't let up just because the baby's out. As levels of estrogen and progesterone plunge, you may come down with a thump, too. Until your hormones settle down and resume normal transmission (honestly, it does happen), it's best to expect a few tears and tantrums—from you, that is, not the baby. OK, it's perfectly normal. It's called the baby blues, and somewhere between half and three-fourths of all new moms get it.

Day three is the humdinger: the initial excitement has waned, you may be almost psychotic with lack of sleep, your tits hurt, and you might be on your own at home, with a new baby and a flood of worries and fears.

Guilt-edged insecurities

Guilt is often a big factor. If you'd planned to have a 100 percent natural home birth, and ended up with an epidural and an emergency Cesarean, you might be battling feelings of failure and inadequacy. In addition, soft-focus photographs of models cradling exquisite babies have skewed our image of motherhood. The reality might seem like an endless cycle of midnight feeds, puke stains, and hunger pangs (you've forgotten to eat, or don't have the energy to cook). Your boobies and belly will have headed south, and the prospect of wearing anything from your prepregnancy wardrobe will be as remote as Uzbekistan. These days, the agony is amplified by paparazzi shots of Hollywood moms who squeeze their bony butts back into size eight jeans before their six-week checkup. Sure, this takes hard work and dedication, but it also takes personal trainers, diet gurus, professional cooks, and a team of nannies to look after baby while mom's pounding the treadmill. Examine your priorities—what's more important, a healthy, happy baby and mom, or a Halle Berry sixpack?—and set yourself attainable goals. These might be limited to getting showered and dressed before 10:00 a.m., and making it to the park every day.

The arsenic hour

You're more likely to feel low at certain times of the day. Some moms call it the arsenic hour, although we're not sure whether you're supposed to take the stuff yourself or give it to your baby. It starts at around 5:00 p.m. or 6:00 p.m., and can go on for a couple of hours. Some people say that babies are miserable at this time of the day because they've accumulated a lot of trapped gas; others say that it's not that the babies are any worse, it's just that by this time the moms are reaching the limits of their endurance. Being aware that it happens is half the battle.

Try to structure your day so that you've got a little time to yourself. Half an hour in the tub, or a catnap in the sun, can make the difference between coping and moping. Don't make the mistake of trying to catch up on all the chores when your baby's asleep, no matter how many disapproving looks your mom-in-law is throwing out. If it worries her that much, show her where the cleaning materials are kept. Even better, get a cleaner, even if it's only for a week or two. When it comes to chores, accept every offer of help, and cut every corner that you can. Washing everything on a warm cycle instead of a hot one is more environmentally friendly, and it also means that there's no need to sort out the whites from the colors. If anyone complains that your whites aren't whiter than white, tell them to get a life.

Just like a pair of jeans, the baby blues will fade. Sometimes it's hard to decide where the blues end and postpartum depression begins, particularly when you're stuck in the middle of an emotional maelstrom. Warning signs include: sleeplessness (lying awake when you've got the chance to sleep, not lack of sleep caused by being up all night with a howling baby); self-esteem that's lower than the GNP in a recession; panic attacks; and confusion. This last doesn't refer to the slightly scatty loss of memory that you might have had during pregnancy, but a big feeling of WHY?—as in, why am I feeling so awful when I should be feeling fulfilled and fantastic? Feeling anger toward your baby is another warning sign (feeling anger toward your mom or mom-in-law is normal). Don't be afraid to ask for help—the longer you stick your head in the sand and pretend there isn't a problem, the worse things will get. Antidepressants might be the shovels you need to dig yourself out of the pit. They're not addictive, they're not going to hurt your baby, and you'll probably need them for only a very short time. You may also want to get your thyroid function checked out, because this is one of the causes of postpartum depression.

WALK IT

Unless temperatures are sub-freezing, ignore any suggestions that you shouldn't take your baby out when it's cold—that's what warm clothing and weatherproof stroller covers are for. There's nothing like a gentle stroll to get a fractious baby to sleep and shake off a mild bout of the blues.

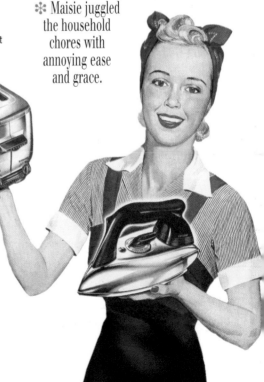

✴ Maisie juggled the household chores with annoying ease and grace.

OOPS, I'VE TURNED INTO A PARENT!

So, you are now officially a parent, and you've got the progeny and paperwork to prove it. Slowly—so slowly that you might not even notice it's happening—things begin to get a little easier. You can change a diaper in under a minute, and can answer many questions, like: why is my baby crying? Shitty diaper, hunger, or gas? You've probably already worked out how to solve the first two (and if you haven't, you're beyond our help).

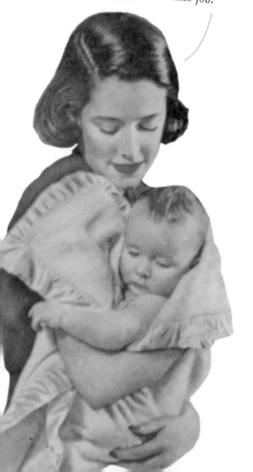

❋ Why did I ever think running the World Bank was a full-time job?

If the classic over-your-shoulder technique doesn't work for gas, try placing the baby, tummy down, across your knees, and stroking its back firmly from the butt up. Other questions will start to arise. Should the baby sleep in our bed? It's fine, so long as you're both happy with the idea. You won't roll over and smother the baby unless you're stoned senseless with booze or drugs, which we don't recommend. Should we let our baby cry? You shouldn't let a newborn cry, but as babies get older there is an argument for what's called "controlled crying"—our moms probably called it "letting them know who's boss." Some people can't bear the thought, or the noise. Read up on both schools, and talk to other parents before making up your mind.

If you're going back to work, start making plans and looking into childcare options as soon as you can. Don't be too horrified if you find that your career suddenly doesn't seem so important any more: priorities change. Parenthood can be a primal affair. It can also be a love affair, and you might start to wonder why it took you so long to get started, and how many more babies you can squeeze into your life (and your house).

Beginnings and endings

In terms of the medical profession, and the guys and gals in white jackets, pregnancy and childbirth come to an end a couple of months after the birth, with your Week Six checkup. By this stage you should have lost around 20 pounds (9 kg), although sometimes the weight doesn't shift until you stop breast-feeding. Your practitioner will check that your uterus has gone back to its normal size; that your cervix is starting to look like its old self again, that any episiotomy or Cesarean scars have healed; and that your blood pressure is back to normal. Your doctor will also discuss what sort of birth control you want to use. Yep, physically speaking, you should be ready for sex. Breast-feeding is not a contraceptive option—or not one that works— and if you used a diaphragm before, you'll need to be refitted. IUDs can also be used if your physician thinks it is suitable. Progestin-only shots or pills can be used while breast-feeding, but you may not like the idea. In fact, you may not like the idea of sex, period. Tiredness can play havoc with your libido, and if you're breast-feeding you may be deficient in estrogen, which can make your vagina a bit drier than usual. Get some lubricants, tell your partner how you're feeling, and start slowly with a bit of mind sex and flirting.

Maybe you can't wait to make a sibling. Try to resist the urge. If you are exclusively breast-feeding you will probably—but not always—stop menstruating, so chances of conceiving are low. It usually takes close to two years for your body to build up its reserves of iron and calcium. In the meantime, you can put into practice all the stuff you've learned about what to avoid and what nutrients you really need (don't forget your calcium and multivitamin intake!).

The Week Six checkup marks the end of your adventure as far as your physician or nurse-midwife is concerned, but for you, and your partner, it's just the beginning of the story. Your baby has probably hit their first important developmental milestone (cracking a smile that's definitely a smile and not a grimace from gas!) but there is a whole lifetime of them ahead. Just don't expect any of them to arrive on schedule. Babies may be many things—wonderful, infuriating, exhausting, fascinating, screaming, gurgling, happy, miserable, adorable, to mention just a few— but they are rarely predictable.

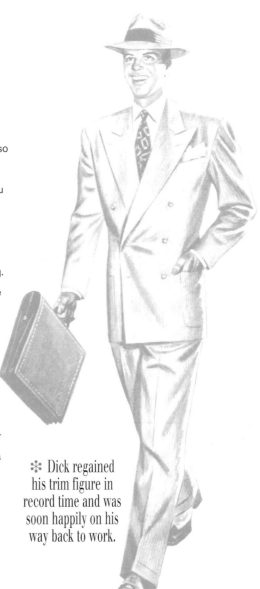

✳ Dick regained his trim figure in record time and was soon happily on his way back to work.

FURTHER READING

What to Expect When You're Expecting

Arlene Eisenberg, Heidi E. Murkoff, and Sandee E. Hathaway

WORKMAN, 2002

The Encyclopedia of Pregnancy and Birth

Janet Balaskas and Yehudi Gordon

TRANS-ATLANTIC PUBLICATIONS, INC., 1989

The Pregnancy Journal: A Day-to-Day Guide to a Healthy and Happy Pregnancy

A. Christine Harris

CHRONICLE BOOKS, 1996

The Girlfriends' Guide to Pregnancy: Or Everything Your Doctor Won't Tell You

Vicky Iovine

POCKET BOOKS, 1995

Butterflies and Hiccups: A Guided Pregnancy Journal

Laurie J. Wing

JAIMCO PUBLISHING, 2002

The Mother of All Pregnancy Books: The Ultimate Guide to Conception, Birth, and Everything In Between

Ann Douglas

JOHN WILEY & SONS, 2002

The Unofficial Guide to Having a Baby

Ann Douglas and John R. Sussman M. D.

JOHN WILEY & SONS, 1999

Pregnancy For Dummies®

Joanne Stone, Keith Eddleman, Mary Murray, and M. D. Stone

JOHN WILEY & SONS, 1999

A Guide to Effective Care in Pregnancy and Childbirth

Marc J. Kirse (ed.), Murray Enkin, Caroline Crowther, James Neilson, Ellen Hodnett, Justus Hofmeyr, and Leila Duley

OXFORD UNIVERSITY PRESS, 2000

The Pregnancy Book: Month-by-Month, Everything You Need to Know From America's Baby Experts

Martha Sears, William Sears, and Linda H. Holt

LITTLE BROWN & CO., 1997

Conception, Pregnancy, and Birth

Miriam Stoppard

DK PUBLISHING, 2000

1000 Questions About Your Pregnancy: Everything Every Expecting Woman Needs to Know

Jeffrey Thurston, M. D.

TAPESTRY PRESS, 2002

Pregnancy and Birth: Your Questions Answered

Christoph C. Lees, Karina Reynolds, and Grainne McCartan

DK PUBLISHING, 2002

Giving Birth

Mary M. Kalergis

SUGARDAY BOOKS, 1997

Your Pregnancy Week By Week

Glade B. Curtis and Judith Schuler

FISHER BOOKS, 2000

The Complete Book of Pregnancy and Childbirth

Sheila Kitzinger and Marcia May

KNOPF, 1996

Preparing for Birth with Yoga: Exercises for Pregnancy and Childbirth

Janet Balaskas

ELEMENT BOOKS, 1994

The Pregnancy Diet: A Healthy Weight Control Program for Pregnant Women

Eileen Behan

POCKET BOOKS, 1999

When You're Expecting Twins, Triplets, or Quads: A Complete Resource

Barbara Luke and Tamara Eberlein

HARPER PERENNIAL, 1999

Deep Relaxation for Childbirth

Dr. Stewart Zelman

CENTERS FOR MOTIVATION, INC., 2001

Preemies: The Essential Guide for Parents of Premature Babies

Dana Wechsler Linden, Emma Trenti Paroli, and Mia Wechsler Doron M. D.

POCKET BOOKS, 2000

This Isn't What I Expected: Overcoming Postpartum Depression

Karen Kleiman and Valerie Davis Raskin

BANTAM BOOKS, 1994

Complete Book of Mother and Baby Care

Canadian Medical Association

READER'S DIGEST ASSOCIATION OF CANADA, 1997

Babies! A Parent's Guide to Surviving and Enjoying Baby's First Year

Dr. Christopher Green

FAWCETT BOOKS, 1994

The Expectant Father: Facts, Tips, and Advice for Dads-To-Be

Armin A. Brott

ABBEVILLE PRESS, INC., 2001

Every Guy's Guide as to What to Expect When She's Expecting

William Grant Eppler, Ruth Davis Barr (ed.)

FURLIP PUBLISHING COMPANY, 2000

A Silent Sorrow: Pregnancy Loss— Guidance and Support for You and Your Family

Ingrid Kohn, Perry-Lynn Moffitt, Isabelle A. Wilkins, Michael R. Berman

ROUTLEDGE, 2000

USEFUL CONTACTS

GENERAL INFORMATION

American Academy of Family Physicians

P.O. Box 11210

Shawnee Mission,

KS 66207-1210

Tel: 800-274-2237 (toll free)

www.aafp.org

American College Of Obstetricians and Gynecologists

409 12th Street

S.W. P.O. BOX 96920

Washington DC 20090-6920

www.acog.org

American Diabetes Association

1701 North Beauregard Street

Alexandria, VA 22311

Tel: 1-800-DIABETES or 1-800-342-2383)

www.diabetes.org

Centers for Medicare & Medicaid Services

7500 Security Boulevard,

Baltimore MD 21244-1850

Tel: 877-267-2323 (toll free)

www.cms.hhs.gov

Child Care Aware

1319 F. Street, NW, Suite 500

Washington, DC 20004

Tel: 800-424-2246 (toll free)

www.childcareaware.org

Internal Revenue Service

Tel: 1-800-829-1040 or

1-800-829-4059 (TDD) for people with hearing impairments

www.irs.gov

March of Dimes

1275 Mamaroneck Ave.,

White Plains, NY 10605

Tel: 914-428-7100

www.marchofdimes.com

National Organization of Single Mothers

www.singlemothers.org

Pre-eclampsia Foundation

P.O. Box 52993

Bellevue, WA 98015-2993

Tel: 425-885-3498 or

1-800-665-9341(toll free)

Email: info@preeclampsia.org

www.preeclampsia.org

Sidelines High-Risk Pregnancy Support

P.O. Box 1808

Laguna Beach, CA 92652

Tel: 888-447-4754 (HI-RISK4)

Email : sidelines@sidelines.org

www.sidelines.org

MOTHER AND BABY'S HEALTH AND NUTRITION

American Dietetic Association

216 W. Jackson Blvd.

Chicago, IL 60606-6995

Tel: 312-899-0040

www.eatright.org

Food and Drug Administration (FDA)

5600 Fishers Lane

Rockville, Maryland 20857

Tel: 1-888-INFO-FDA / 1-888-463-6332 for general inquiries

www.fda.com

Maternal and Child Health Bureau

Parklawn Building Room 18-05

5600 Fishers Lane, Rockville,

Maryland 20857

Tel: 301-443-2216

www.mchb.hrsa.gov

National Institute of Child Health and Human Development

Bldg 31,

Room 2A32, MSC 2425

31 Center Drive

Bethesda, MD 20892-2425

Tel: 800-370-2943

www.nichd.nih.gov

National Women's Health Information Center

Department of Health and Human Services

200 Independence Avenue, SW

Room 730B

Washington, DC 20201

Tel: 202-690-7650

Breast-feeding helpline: 1-800-994-WOMAN (9662)

www.4women.gov

USDA Center for Nutrition Policy and Promotion

1120 20th Street NW

Suite 200, North Lobby

Washington, DC 20036

Tel: 202-606-8000

www.usda.gov/cnpp

CHILDBIRTH INFORMATION

American Academy of Husband-coached Childbirth

P.O. Box 5224

Sherman Oaks, CA 91413-5224

Tel: 800/4-A-BIRTH

or 818/788-6662

www.bradleybirth.com

American College of Nurse-Midwives

818 Connecticut Avenue, NW,

Suite 900

Washington DC 20006

Tel: 202-728-9860

www.midwife.org

Association of Labor Assistants and Childbirth Educators

P.O. Box 390436

Cambridge, MA 02139

Tel: 617-441-2500

www.alace.org

Doulas of North America

PO Box 626

Jasper, IN 47547

Tel: 888-788-DONA or 812-634-1491

Referral line: 801-756-7331

E-mail: Referrals@DONA.org

www.dona.org

International Cesarean Awareness Network

www.ican-online.org

International Childbirth Education Association, Inc.

P.O. Box 20048

Minneapolis, Minnesota 55420

Tel: 952-854-8660

.www.icea.org

Lamaze International

2025 M Street, Suite 800,

Washington DC 20036-3309

Tel: 202-367-1128

www.lamaze.org

Midwives Alliance Of North America

4805 Lawrenceville Hwy

Suite 116-279

Lilburn, GA 30047

Tel: 888-923-MANA (6262)

E-mail info@mana.org

www.mana.org

National Association of Childbearing Centers

3123 Gottschall Road,

Perkiomenville, Pennsylvania 18074

Tel: 215-234-8068

E-mail: ReachNACC@BirthCenters.org

www.birthcenters.org

BREAST-FEEDING

La Leche League

1400 N. Meacham Road,

Schaumburg, IL 60173-4808

Tel 847-519-7730

www.lalecheleague.org

Medela, Inc.

1101 Corporate Dr.,

McHenry, IL 60050

Tel: 1-800-435-8316

www.medela.com

Wellstart International

P.O. Box 80877

San Diego, California 92138-0877

Tel: 619-295-5192

Helpline: 619-295-5192

E-mail: info@wellstart.org

www.wellstart.org

MULTIPLE BIRTHS

Center for Loss in Multiple Birth Inc.

c/o Jean Kollantai, P.O. Box 91377,

Anchorage, AK 99509

Tel: 907-222-5321

Email: newsletter@climb-support.org

www.climb-support.org

Center for the Study of Multiple Births

Suite 464,

333 East Superior Street,

Chicago, IL 60611

Tel: 1-312-908-7532

www.multiplebirth.com

Mothers of Supertwins

P.O. Box 951

Brentwood, NY 11717-0627

Tel: 631-859-1110

E-mail: info@MOSTonline.org

www.mostonline.org

National Organization of Mothers of Twins Clubs Inc.

P.O. Box 438

Thompsons Station,

TN 37179-0438

Tel: 615-595-0936

Email: INFO@nomotc.org

www.nomotc.org

The Triplet Connection

P.O. Box 99571

Stockton, CA 95209

Tel: 209-474-0885

www.tripletconnection.org

Twins Foundation

P.O. Box 6043

Providence,

RI 02940-6043

Tel: 401-729-8946 (Voice)

www.twinsfoundation.com

PREMATURE BABIES

American Association for Premature Infants

P.O. Box 46371

Cincinnati, OH 45246-0371

Tel: 513-956-4331

www.aapi-online.org

BABIES WITH SPECIAL
NEEDS/BIRTH DEFECTS
American Cleft Palate-
Craniofacial
Association/Cleft Palate
Foundation

104 South Estes Drive,

Suite 204, Chapel Hill,

NC 27514

Tel: 919-933-9044

www.cleftline.org

Family Voices National
Office (support for children with
special needs)

3411Candelaria NE, Suite M

Albuquerque, NM 87107

Tel: 505-872-4774 or

1-888-835-5669 (toll free)

www.familyvoices.org

National Down
Syndrome Society

666 Broadway,

New York, NY 10012

Tel: 212-460-9330 or

800-221-4602 (toll free)

Email: info@ndss.org

www.ndss.org

National Information Center
for Children and Youth with
Disabilities

P.O. Box 1492

Washington DC 20013

Tel: 800-695-0285

www.nichcy.org

National Organization
for Rare Disorders

55 Kenosia Avenue

PO Box 1968

Danbury, CT 06813-1968

Tel: -203-744-0100 or (800) 999-6673 (toll free—voicemail only)

www.rarediseases.org

POSTNATAL INFORMATION
Allergy & Asthma Network
Mothers of Asthmatics

2751 Prosperity Ave., Suite 150

Fairfax, VA 22031

Tel: 800-878-4403

www.aanma.org

Depression After
Delivery, Inc.

91 East Somerset Street

Raritan, NJ 08869

Tel: 1-800-944-4773 (4PPD)

(Information Request Line)

www.depressionafterdelivery.com

SAFETY INFORMATION
The Danny Foundation

Tel: 1-800-83DANNY

Email: info@dannyfoundation.org

www.dannyfounation.org

SafetyBeltSafe U.S.A.

P. O. Box 553

Altadena, CA 91003

www.carseat.org

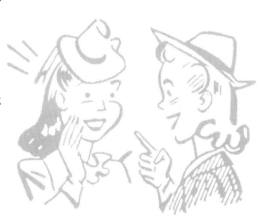

INDEX

ACKNOWLEDGMENTS

Thank you to everyone who helped with the creation of this book, particularly Caroline, Viv, and the many moms who shared their stories. But most of all, I'd like to thank my husband—and soulmate—Kevin for all his support, encouragement, and, above all, patience. Without him, none of this would have been possible. He has also given me the greatest gift of all—two wonderful children, Lydia and Alistair.

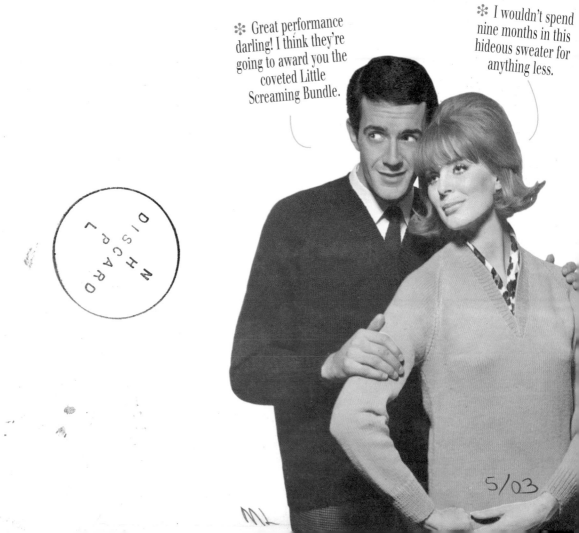